Your metabolism: a user's guide

Knowing the biochemistry of the human body to be fitter, healthier and thinner

Simon Windsor

Introduction

"I can't stand people who do not take food seriously."
Oscar Wilde

The attempt to search for the word "diet" on a popular online bookstore opens up a world of revolutionary programs. Limited to the first results from tens of thousands of titles present, we have: the diet of super metabolism, the diet of longevity, the paleo diet, the protein diet, the diet of hormones, the vegan diet, the smart-food diet, the fasting diet, the smart diet, the diet of blood groups, the ketogenic diet, the diet without mucus, the green detox diet, the anti-inflammatory diet, the alkaline diet, the genetic diet, the water diet, the Mediterranean diet, the nutritarian diet, the low carb diet, the deception of the low carb diets, the super-health diet, the happy bowel diet, the flexible diet, the mental diet, the super-food diet, etc.

There is something weird: in the history of mankind, there has never been a maniacal attention to what we eat that is equal to that of our time. And, if you think about it, being able to easily get diverse foods has never been easier. Your great-grandfather didn't have the chance to taste goji berries. Likely, he had problems getting meat every day.

On the other hand, however, the diseases associated with poor nutrition are like a biblical catastrophe almost unknown in other eras: a recent FAO report shows that within roughly ten years, one in three people in the world will suffer from food-related issues: obesity, diabetes, cardiovascular disease, and cancer. And as we get closer to our daily lives, many of us struggle to keep our weight under control and get easily tired, anxious and without energy. Furthermore, many even age early despite trying to eat (more or less) healthily... almost as if their bodies were not forgiving the slightest cheat.

What happened to our relationship with food? Can we say that it has become ill, amidst super-chef reality shows, food fashions that last a few seasons, organic markets with absurd prices and waves of colored junk foods? Why do the diets listed above contradict each other, yet each of them sells itself as the absolute truth?

Maybe we need to draw a line and start over. Our bodies live by an impressive series of chemical reactions; everything we are, feel, and become comes from them. The food we ingest is not burned in a furnace like wood, but is transformed into thousands of molecules that flood our blood and react with our body.

Fattening, slimming, getting old, getting sick, feeling tired... they are simply consequences of these reactions. For this reason, this book aims to understand how our diet should really be structured to keep us healthy, thin, and healthy, but starting from how our body works, and how, from a scientific point of view, different types of food and diet can have different effects on us.

"Scientific" is a key word: we believe that what distinguishes hoaxes from truth is precisely scientific research; in fact, every statement made in the book is accompanied by a reference to a text, study, or scientific article. The material listed can, among other things, be an excellent starting point for those who want to deepen the concepts expressed.

At the same time, we did everything we could to avoid boring our readers to death and making them feel as if they were sitting, half-asleep, at a long conference. All the concepts, in fact, are expressed in a simple way, suitable also for those who, in their lives, deal with something entirely different. We have also tried to enrich the various themes as much as possible with anecdotes and true stories. The illustrations that accompany the text, finally, allow us to visualize the concepts in a far more immediate and entertaining form.

The ambition of this book, therefore, is not to be yet another work on the miraculous diet for a spectacular body or for living a hundred years eating only this and that food, but a way to understand, in a scientific but enjoyable way, how our body and our metabolism work and, only in relation to this, which foods should be consumed and in what quantities. We will go so far as to give readers the tools to build their own balanced diet based on their own needs; the knowledge that we will use for this purpose will be built step by step in the different chapters.

After reading this book, you will know more about your body and nutrition than 99 percent of the people around you know, and you will be able to independently distinguish hoaxes from truth, understand what has a scientific foundation and what does not. Above all, you will have all the tools to manage your diet independently, not only to reach your ideal weight, but also to live more and feel more energetic, healthy and (why not) beautiful than you ever were. You can be your own dietician.

This is how our path is structured:

- The first part of the book begins with the basics, introducing the protagonists. We will meet the various substances that make up foods and their functions beyond the platitudes that are normally proposed
- The second part addresses the issue of metabolism, trying to understand how our body manages each of these substances, why, and with what effects
- The third part uses all the accumulated knowledge, plus other studies, to give you the tools needed to build your own healthy eating habits to preserve and improve your health and energy. In addition, it provides the theoretical and practical knowledge to build a real diet adapted to your specific needs in terms of body weight
- The fourth part completes the journey where the journey of food also ends: in our intestines, with what is not digested, and with the last frontiers on its relationship with health

We hope that this will be a fascinating journey for all and that it will help spread a concept: scientific research must be the only source of the statements that circulate: only by relying on what is proven and demonstrable can we improve, in indisputable terms, our appearance, our health, and our lives.

PART ONE

The Biochemistry of Food

1. Proteins and Amino Acids

"We are a fearsome mixture of nucleic acids and memories, desires and proteins".
François Jacob

The First Soup in History

When we hear about protein, we think of something that is contained in steak and beans, and that seems to be very fashionable among health-conscious people. As a matter of fact, proteins are much more than the piece of tuna that we should add to our salad following the latest Californian diet: they are the basis of everything that is alive.

Any living thing is made up of proteins: from your mother-in-law to the grass in your garden; from the neighbor's cat to the mosquito that is buzzing around you. Proteins are, in fact, the main bricks that form all living cells; we need them for the continuous processes of repairs and replacements taking place in our bodies. Imagine a city: there will always be a need for new bricks, because there will always be buildings to replace, expand, or refine.

But the function of proteins goes far beyond that. Some of them, more than bricks, are real gears: they perform irreplaceable tasks within living beings. It is a protein that makes our hearts beat faster when we are excited; it is a protein that allows us to digest food; it is a protein that heals us from the flu; it is a protein that makes us tanned; and it is a protein that makes us enjoy having sex or biting a piece of chocolate. These are just a few examples; in practically everything that happens to you during the day, be sure, a different protein is involved.

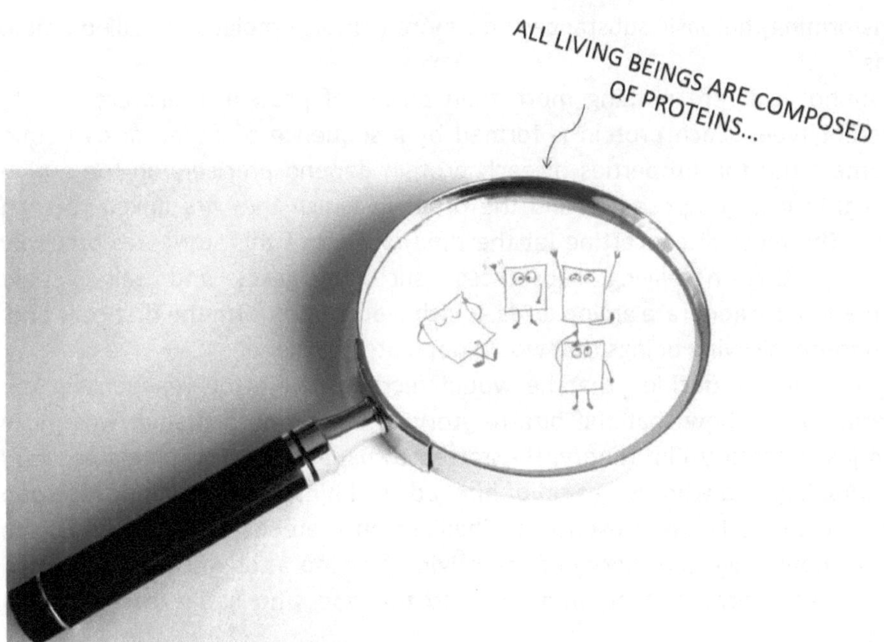

It is therefore worth starting our journey right here. And to do that, we have to go back in time by many, many millennia. Four billion years ago... an amount of time that's hard to even imagine. Our planet was much less hospitable than it is today at the time: continuous earthquakes, gigantic volcanic explosions, rivers of incandescent lava, extreme weather conditions and poisonous air; not exactly the ideal place for a relaxing holiday. There was, of course, still no trace of any kind of living creatures.

In 1953, the experiment of a young assistant at the University of Chicago caused a real sensation. Stanley Miller, then 23, was very impressed by the science fiction theories of Nobel Prize winner Harold Urey during a university seminar. Urey, drawing on some of the theories that had been circulating since the 1920s, talked about how, precisely in the extreme environment of the primordial earth, the adventure of life could have begun. Loose in the water of newborn oceans, Urey explained, salts and other basic chemical compounds were very common (in the scientific world this ancient mixture has the suggestive name of "primordial soup"). The lightning energy of the many thunderstorms could have caused various chemical reactions in this soup, transforming the basic substances into more complex molecules, called amino acids.

Amino acids are nothing more than pieces of protein; there are twenty different types. Each protein is formed by a sequence of amino acids bound together, and the properties of each protein depend precisely on the amino acids that it is composed of and the order in which they are linked to each other. The most disconcerting (at the time) aspect of this story was precisely the fact that non-living substances, such as gases and salts, could spontaneously generate amino acids, which would later form the first cells and, from there, all living beings that would populate the planet.

Young Miller decided that he would recreate the same reactions in the laboratory, to show that the bizarre story of the primordial soup was more than just a fantasy film theory. He started to badger Urey, who was not very encouraging, and who, to get rid of him, advised him to forget about the soup and instead study the presence of Thallium on meteorites (this gives us the idea of how much the theory of the origin of amino acids must have seemed exotic and bizarre at that time, even to the one who had exposed it in a seminar!).

But the stubborn Miller did not give in: he became so adamant until Urey, exhausted, agreed to support him in his experiment.

Miller inserted into a glass sphere the main elements that were supposed to be part of the primordial soup: water, hydrogen, ammonia and methane. Then he constantly applied various electric shocks to simulate the frequent lightning strikes of the young earth. "During the experiment," says Miller, "the water turned pale pink on the first day. At the end of the week it turned red and turbid." Analyzing the content of that foul-smelling liquid, Miller exulted: it was really amino acids! [1]

[1] *Miller S. L., Production of Amino Acids Under Possible Primitive Earth Conditions (PDF), in Science, 117(3046), 1953, pp. 528-529,* DOI:10.1126/science.117.3046.528.

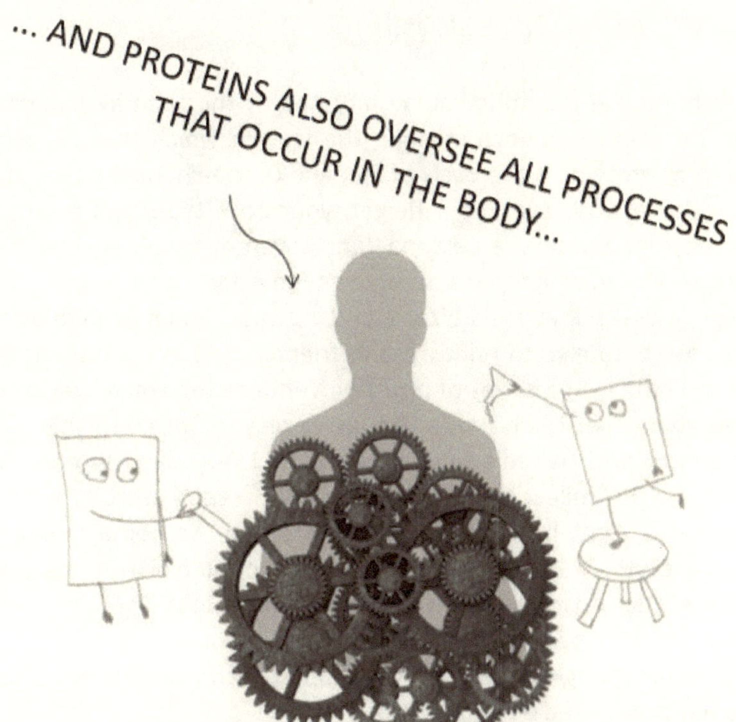

The guy's stubbornness was rewarded: the prestigious Time dedicated an article to him with the disconcerting title: "Semi-Creation". The experiment had, in fact, greatly impressed both the scientific community and ordinary people, because for the first time it was shown that inert matter could be transformed into the basis of proteins, and therefore of living beings. "Professor Urey and student Miller," wrote the article, "do not think they have created life. What they did was to demonstrate that the complex organic compounds found in living matter can be formed, through chemical reactions, from gases that were probably common in the primordial earth's atmosphere. If their experimental apparatus had continued to simulate those conditions for years, rather than just a week, it could have created something like the first living molecule."

The Inventor in the Landfill

The excitement the scientific community had at the time in clarifying the origin of amino acids is understandable: the way in which these substances combine to form proteins is the basis of life, and of the characteristics of living beings. The color of your eyes, your height, your body type, and even part of your personality depend on the personal (and different from any other human being on earth!) way in which you assemble amino acids.

This is how it works: imagine a bizarre and ingenious old man with a passion for building objects to give to relatives and friends. He has a whole notebook with the design details of a series of bizarre inventions he would like to create: a cat-shaped chandelier for his wife, a toaster playing music for his nephew and a refrigerator with wheels for his neighbor. Every day, he goes to the municipal landfill to collect everything that may seem useful to him: old washing machines, light bulbs, car parts, and so on. At home, he carefully disassembles everything until he gets to the most basic pieces: screws, wires, microchips, gaskets, resistances and pieces of sheet metal. Then he opens his notebook and carefully begins to assemble his creations.

Finally, all triumphant, he gives the cat-shaped chandelier to his better half (who would have preferred a diamond ring).

Your body does, more or less, the same thing with proteins. It carefully disassembles the proteins we eat (the items collected at the landfill) until it gets to their essential components: the amino acids. Then it recombines them to form what it needs (all the specific proteins you need). The basic constituents are always the same, only the way in which they are assembled changes. The notebook with the instructions is our DNA, the precious code contained in all our cells, which gives them the instructions to assemble the amino acids into proteins. If our DNA says that your eyes are blue, then proteins are produced to color your iris in this way. If it says that you are tall and lanky, proteins are produced, which tend to put together bones and tissues in that way. Think about it next time you eat a steak: after being broken down into microscopic units, that meat will be re-assembled to form your muscles, your bones or your hair, according to the instructions that your personal and unique DNA will give.

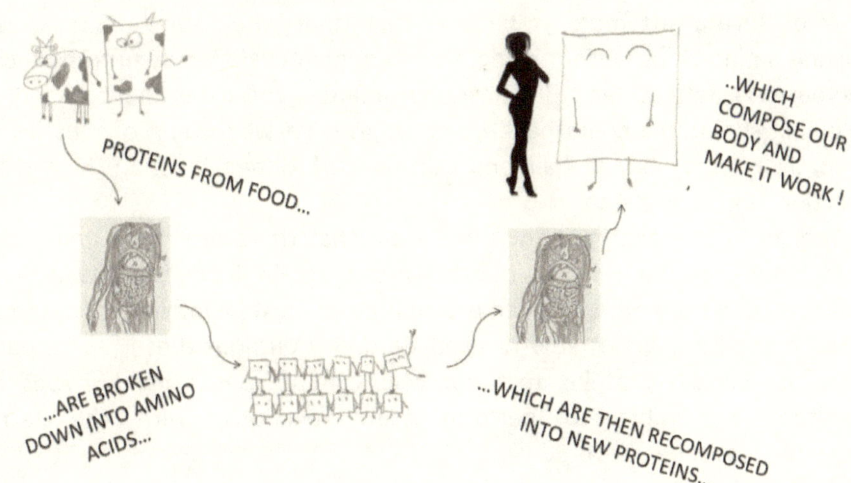

However, not all of the pieces the old man collects from the landfill are the same. If he lacks a piece of sheet metal, he can always obtain it from something else; for instance, he can melt a piece of metal and then beat it with a hammer like a blacksmith. But there are some pieces that are really irreplaceable: for instance, despite all his good will, he is not really able to produce a microchip from something else. Back to our body: do we need to introduce ALL the amino acids with food?

The Poor Students of Professor William

In the 1940s, the American biochemist William Cumming Rose conducted an experiment to answer this question[2]. He proposed a very special diet to some of his volunteer students (who hopefully received at least a higher grade for the inconvenience). The bases of the meals were, in fact, foods low in protein, but providing all the other necessary nutrients: corn starch, sugar, butter, corn oil, salts and vitamins. Separately, the students received rations of purified amino acids. In this way, Rose could precisely control which amino acids the students were or were not receiving each time, and the effects on their health.

---

[2] *William C. Rose*. "Feeding experiments with mixtures of highly purified amino acids: I. The inadequacy of diets containing nineteen amino acids" *(PDF). The Journal of Biological Chemistry 94: 155–165.*

After several attempts, it became clear that when some of the twenty existing amino acids were missing, the students developed symptoms such as nervousness, fatigue, and dizziness. Fortunately, the experiment ended: the following symptoms could have been progressive weakening of muscles and strength, edema, loss of hair and skin, loss of kidney function, high risk of infection, and even death.

Thanks to this experiment, it was clear that there are some amino acids (called non-essential), which our body can obtain from other substances. However, there are others (called essential) that must be introduced with food, because our body is not able to produce them. Without these "spare parts", there are certain proteins that our cells can no longer build. It becomes therefore impossible to perform their functions, with the terrible consequences seen above.

Of the 20 amino acids that make up all proteins, 8 are essential, 10 are non-essential, and two are essential only in childhood. The names of the essential amino acids could be those that an alien would give to his pets: Phenylalanine, Leucine, Threonine, Tryptophan, Valine, Isoleucine, Methionine, Lysine.

It is therefore mandatory, if we want to remain healthy and allow our body to function properly, to take all eight essential amino acids from foods containing them[3].

Here are the main foods that contain the essential amino acids:

•   Phenylalanine: legumes (especially beans, chickpeas, lentils, broad beans); cheese, eggs, rabbit meat, wheat, peanuts and avocado. It is also found in some synthetic sweeteners.

•   Leucine: cereals, dried fruit, legumes, chicken, cheese and fish.

•   Threonine: legumes (especially chickpeas and peas), dried fruit, and mushrooms.

•   Tryptophan: bananas, milk and dairy products, oats, dates, meat, peanuts, eggs, legumes, fish, sesame seeds and chocolate.

•   Valine: legumes (especially broad beans, peas and lentils), dried fruit, lamb and pork meat, fish (especially salmon) and cheese.

•   Isoleucine: beef, lamb and chicken meat; sardines, cheese, lentils, soya, eggs, almonds and peanuts.

---

[3] *Young VR (1994). "Adult amino acid requirements: the case for a major revision in current recommendations" (PDF). J. Nutr. 124 (8 Suppl): 1517S–1523S. PMID 8064412.*

- Methionine: fish, whole grains, dairy products (especially hard cheese) and some seaweeds.

- Lysine: soya, legumes, cod, sardines, chicken, pork, red meat and cheese.

We have also mentioned two amino acids that are considered essential only in childhood. These are arginine (dried fruit, legumes, meat, fish, cheese and eggs) and histidine (legumes, pork, cereals containing gluten, wheat germ and peanuts).

Including these foods in a varied way within one's diet is therefore a guarantee of good health. This does not mean that we have to get anxious ("Quick, a sardine! I'm afraid I'm deficient in isoleucine!"): in general, non-vegetarians take all the essential amino acids from foods of animal origin such as meat, fish and eggs without any problems (the proteins contained in these foods are called "nobles" precisely because they have a very complete amino acid profile). However, as you can see from the list of foods, variety is important. Eating chicken breast every day as the only source of protein leads, in the long run, to a situation of deficiency.

There is also good news for vegetarians and vegans: even if the proteins contained in plant foods do not have all the essential amino acids together (they are not "noble"), it is possible to obtain a complete amino acid profile by combining various plant sources. By regularly eating cereals and legumes, and perhaps supplementing with dried fruit, for instance, you will take all the eight essential amino acids. It is also clear that any diet or feeding regime that deprives our body of the foods above for long periods is harmful, no discussion![4].

---

[4] Dietary Reference Intakes: The Essential Guide to Nutrient Requirements. Institute of Medicine's Food and Nutrition Board. usda.gov

2.Vitamins and Mineral Salts

"Pop music is aspirin and the blues are vitamins"
Peter Tork

Cartier and the Wizard

We are in Canada, near Montreal. It is the freezing winter of 1535, and the waters of the Saint Lawrence river have turned into ice, blocking three sailing ships. These are the ships of Jacques Cartier's expedition, sent by the King of France to seek gold in the new world. But something more frightening than glacial temperatures threatens the crew: of the 110 sailors, 25 have already died, and almost all the others are seriously ill. It is scurvy, the nightmare of the seafarers of the past.

It often happened that entire crews, during the interminable crossing of the oceans, began to experience increasingly serious symptoms: wounds that opened spontaneously in the skin, bleeding gums, ulcers, tremendous joint pain. The skin would become yellowish, dry, and sometimes cover itself with horrible swelling and stains.

Cartier's crew, and perhaps himself, would have been doomed to death if it had not been for a local Indian tribe, the Iroquois, with whom (luckily for him) Cartier had been kind and very friendly.

The chief of the Iroquois visited the battered crew and recognized the presence of evil spirits, who sometimes took possession of his men as well. The only way to cast them out, he explained, was to drink the liquid obtained by boiling the leaves of a sacred tree that the Indians called "annedda". Although reluctant, Cartier followed the advice of the Indian chief, and all his crew miraculously healed in a short time[5].

It took a few millennia before Western medicine was able to provide a scientific response to the history of evil spirits. It was in 1910, in fact, that the Japanese scientist Umetaro Suzuki isolated from rice bran a new nutrient, the first vitamin. In the following decades twelve more followed, named after

---

[5] *Martini E (2002). "Jacques Cartier witnesses a treatment for scurvy". Vesalius. 8 (1): 2–6. PMID 12422875.*

different letters of the alphabet. The potion of the Iroquois Indians was evidently rich in vitamin C, whose deficiency causes scurvy, which was linked to the poor diet of the crews during long crossings.

Each vitamin is different, but they all have two fundamental elements in common: they are essential for life and our bodies cannot produce them on their own (we must therefore take them necessarily through food). This is not the case for all living beings: as far as vitamin C is concerned, for instance, only man, some monkeys, guinea pigs and some bats have to take it with food. All others produce it themselves. Most likely, when our ancestors lived in the forests, the abundance of vegetables and fruit provided them with all the vitamin C they needed. As a consequence, this led to an evolutionary mutation which no longer produced that substance, releasing energy at the cellular level for other processes[6].

Each vitamin has a specific field of action in our body, which involves different and complex chemical reactions. To give you an idea, let's see what happened inside the bodies of the poor sailors stuck in the Canadian ice.

A Braid Impossible to Make

Collagen is a protein present in abundance in our body, which serves primarily to "fill" and "hold together" our organs and various tissues. This protein, to perform this function, must clearly have a very robust structure. If you take three threads and twist them together while continuing to turn them, you will get a much stronger kind of rope. The structure of the collagen is the same: it is three strands of amino acids twisted together to form a strong "rope" that can hold together our fragile internal organs and tissues.

In order for each of these filaments to take on this "twisted" form, it is necessary that one of the amino acids composing it (called proline) is transformed by the cells of our body into a slightly modified version: hydroxyproline. And in the chemical reaction that transforms proline into hydroxyproline, vitamin C is fundamental[7].

---

[6] PAULING, L.: Evolution and the need for ascorbic acid. Proc. Nat. Acad. Sc. 67:1643-1648, 1970.

[7] Myllylä, R.; Majamaa, K.; Günzler, V.; Hanauske-Abel, H. M.; Kivirikko, K. I. (1984). "Ascorbate is consumed stoichiometrically in the uncoupled reactions catalyzed by propyl 4-hydroxylase and lysyl hydroxylase". *J. Biol. Chem.* 259 (9): 5403–5. PMID 6325436

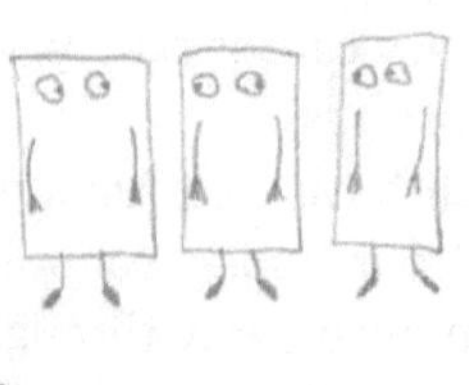

1

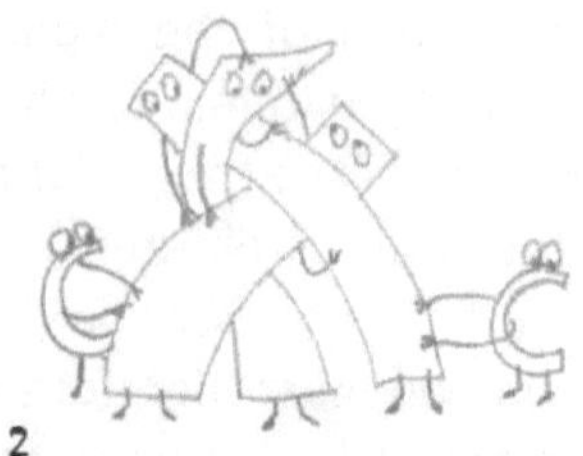

2

COLLAGEN CAN ONLY TAKE ON ITS CHARACTERISTIC FORM THANKS TO VITAMIN C

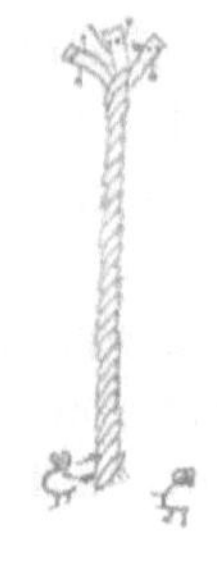

3

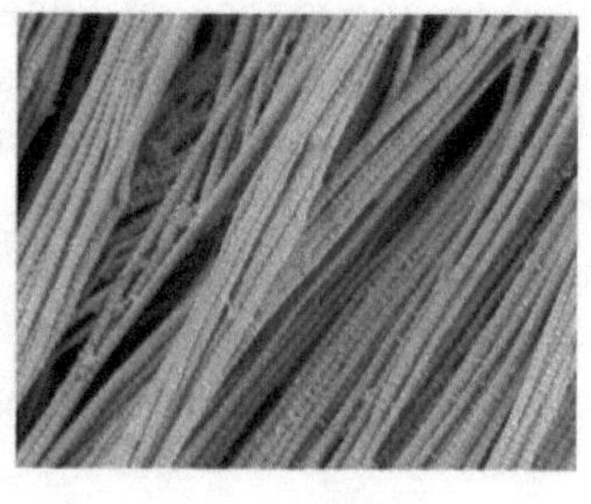

4

So, here's what happened to the sailors: Due to their vitamin C-free diet, their body cells were unable to transform the amino acid proline into the hydroxyproline version. Without hydroxyproline, the collagen molecules could not assume their twisted form (it was like trying to make a braid with dry branches...), and consequently the collagen was much more unstable. The lack of collagen to hold the internal tissues together led to the appearance of blood stains and edemas.

Of course, the tasks of vitamin C do not end here. Each vitamin is multitasking and is therefore involved in a multitude of different reactions. As an example, it is known in popular culture that vitamin C itself helps to strengthen the immune system. This is confirmed by a series of processes at the cellular level: vitamin C increases the production of interferons (proteins produced by a cell attacked by a virus, which increase the resistance of neighboring cells), promotes the multiplication of white blood cells (the defenders of our body), and so on[8].

We don't want to bore you to death here with a detailed description of all the chemical processes related to the various vitamins, but we think a short

---

[8] Med Monatsschr Pharm. 2009 Feb;32(2):49-54; quiz 55-6., [Vitamin C and immune function].Ströhle A[1], Hahn A.

guide of their functions, of the deficiency symptoms and of the foods containing them may be useful. You can find it at the end of the book in Appendix A.

We recommend taking a look especially at the various foods that are rich in different vitamins. Once again, there is no need to go crazy with juices of eighty different vegetables: the important thing is to have the richest and most varied diet possible. If you eat fresh food every day, and if you vary your choice, you should theoretically be protected from the lack of vitamins.

Why did we write "theoretically"? The above sentence would have been absolutely correct in the fifties of the last century, but today it is a little less so. The fact is that plant products are getting poorer in their content of nutrients (vitamins first and foremost).

A study carried out in 2004[9] compared the content of certain nutrients in 43 different types of common plants between 1950 and 1999. The results showed a dramatic decline in nutritional properties; for instance, vitamin B2 had decreased by 38% compared to the past. The same trend was confirmed by several other studies; to name just one[10], the analysis of the differences between foods bought in Canadian supermarkets between 1951 and 1999 showed, for instance, that potatoes had lost almost all of vitamin A and almost 60% of vitamin C, and that consumers would have to eat eight oranges to get the same amount of vitamin C that their grandparents had from just one of those fruits...

What's happening? Is this an occult conspiracy to give everyone scurvy?

Stench and vitamins

The loss of vitamins has gone hand in hand with the disappearance of the stench of the countryside. The fields of the past, in summer, were saturated with the intoxicating aroma of horse and cow poop: farmers used it to grow strong and nutritious plants. The mineral salts naturally present in this fetid brown substance, absorbed by the roots of the plants together with water, are

---

[9] Changes in USDA food composition data for 43 garden crops, 1950 to 1999. Davis DR1, Epp MD, Riordan HD. J Am Coll Nutr. 2004 Dec;23(6):669-82.

[10] Picard, Andre'. "Today's fruits, vegetables lack yesterday's nutrition." Globe & Mail Toronto, ON, Canada, July 6, 2002, A1

in fact the basis of numerous biochemical reactions, including those from which vitamins originate.

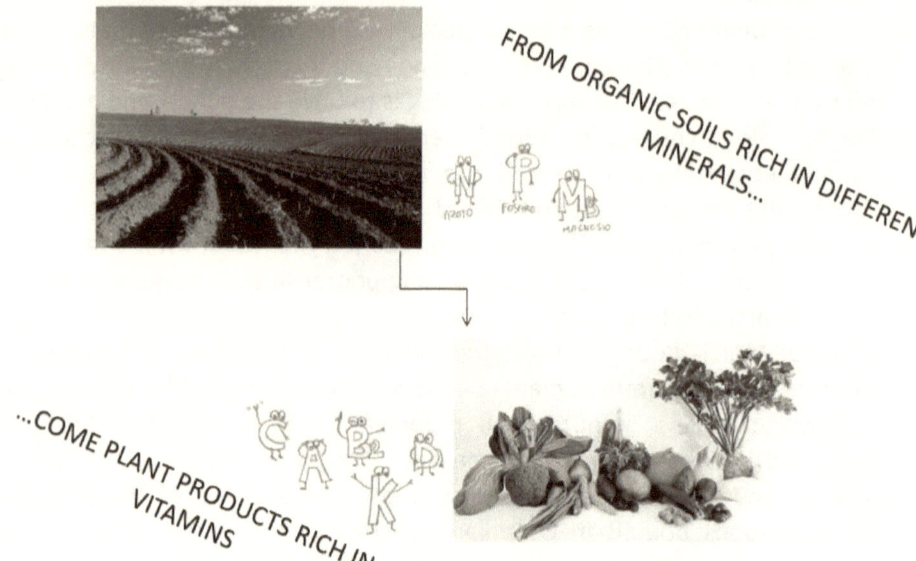

Since the Second World War, synthetic fertilizers have progressively replaced those of animal origin. The countryside smells much better, but lost something. Synthetic fertilizers, in fact, are composed of the three main minerals that the plant kingdom needs: nitrogen, potassium and phosphorus. However, they often lack a multitude of other minerals (such as calcium, magnesium, sulfur, chlorine...) connected to the production of vitamins. It is like coloring a drawing with only red, blue and yellow: you can do it, but the result is certainly not the best possible.

To make matters worse, other factors contributed, such as the use of pesticides and pollution, as well as the intensification of agriculture.

What can we do about this (not being able, of course, to fertilize the fields in place of the horses...)?

First of all, we can obviously try to make up for quality with quantity. It's a good idea to include plenty of fruit, vegetables and the other vitamin-rich fresh foods listed in Appendix A in our diet.

Also, there is a good chance that vegetables and fruits certified as organic will come from fields with cultivation techniques more similar to those of the past (crop rotation, natural fertilizers, focus on product quality rather than on quantity and speed), and will therefore be richer in vitamins.

Transporting agricultural products on long journeys is another cause of the impoverishment in vitamins: it is always better to buy at local organic products markets. If you buy organic products at the supermarket, instead, it may be worth taking a look at the manufacturer's website, to see if there is information on how they treat their crops.

In addition, it is always better to prefer seasonal fruits and vegetables. Besides being tastier, they are more likely to have grown naturally. Frozen vegetables can also be OK: the extreme cold "freezes on the spot" the nutrients of products that are often harvested in their season.

If, in addition, you want to take a multivitamin to make sure you get all the vitamins you need, that will not hurt. It is clear that the primary source of vitamins must be food, but given the importance of these substances, and considering the fact that foods are increasingly poor, it is not a bad idea to take a supplement in moderation.

Every year, among other things, new discoveries are made about vitamins and their properties (for instance, their role in cancer prevention is a very topical issue); therefore, it cannot be excluded that there are benefits that we do not yet know. However, a twentieth-century city in Europe or the United States should be very different from a ship trapped in ice in Canada. How is it possible that, in the era of smartphones, vitamin deficiency could still be an issue?

During a conference of researchers in Italy[11], in 2015, a fairly disconcerting figure was made known: 80% of the population of the country is deficient in vitamin D. The growing number of cases of osteoporosis, and probably also degenerative diseases (such as Alzheimer's and Parkinson's) would be linked to this deficiency.

Even in our developed world, therefore, problems related to vitamin deficiency are present. So, we should not take these eclectic substances for granted: they can make a difference to our quality of life... and perhaps even save it.

Mineral salts differ from vitamins in that they are inorganic compounds, i.e. carbon-free. Like vitamins, mineral salts have essential functions for the life of

---

[11] "Hypovitaminosis D - clinical manifestations and related correlated pathologies", group of interventions coordinated by Carlo Foresta

the body; in Appendix B at the end of the book you can see a list of the salts our body needs, the foods that are rich in them and the main functions they perform. Compared to other nutrients, the daily need for mineral salts is minimal. But, since they are continuously eliminated with sweat, urine and feces, once again a rich and varied diet is the key to get all of them.

3.Fats

"And I believe that if I eat a tub of butter, and no one sees me, the calories
don't count"
Dr. Isobel 'Izzie' Stevens (Katherine Heigl), Grey's Anatomy

Fats are ugly, dirty and bad, aren't they?

How much of this is true? Is that bacon really trying to kill us?

Lipids, or fats, are one of the main organic compounds that allow life, but their reputation in our society is terrible. Let's get to know them better for a little more clarity.

The Secret of Pioppi

Pioppi is a small Italian village of about three hundred inhabitants, not far from Naples. It has wonderful beaches, a blue sea and a picturesque castle. But it is also connected to a modern revolution that has affected the whole world.

The American biologist Ancel Keys settled in this picturesque village in 1962. Fascinated by the low incidence of cardiovascular diseases in southern Italy, he decided to move the headquarters of his studies to a place where he could experience the lifestyle of the locals.

Having probably realized that a life full of sun, sea and fresh fish was not so bad, Keys stayed in Pioppi for forty years, the rest of his life. The conclusions he reached (a diet based on legumes, extra-virgin olive oil, bread, pasta, vegetables, fruit, fish and very little meat was responsible for the beneficial effect on the local population) are now globally known as the Mediterranean diet.

If fats had a deadly enemy, this would be Keys. The studies on the Italian population are in fact part of a larger cycle of analysis started in the fifties, called "Seven Countries Study", which compared the eating habits of about 12,000 people in seven countries (Italy, Holland, Yugoslavia, USA, Finland, Japan and Greece). The result revealed to the world that the number of deaths from heart attacks was much lower among the Mediterranean populations than, for instance, in the Anglo-Saxon and Northern European countries where the diet was rich, alas, in fats (red meat, butter, whole milk and lard)[12].

Keys' studies earned him a cover in the prestigious Times and marked the beginning of fat demonization. From the sixties to the nineties, the Western world took a huge crusade against everything that contained fat: red meat, eggs, even olive oil had suddenly become poison. Supermarket shelves were filled with "light", "skimmed", "diet" and "low-fat" products, and the basis of the so-called "food pyramid" became carbohydrates, as a fat-free food was needed to replace everything that had been branded as unhealthy.

The president of the National Academy of Sciences, Philip Handler, in 1980, declared: "We are embarking on a huge nutritional experiment".

Many voices today argue that the experiment has failed[13]. In the Western world, in fact, in recent decades people are on average much fatter; cardiovascular disease and heart attack continue to be a major cause of death and type two diabetes has increased by 166% since the 1980s. Apparently, the demonization of fats in favor of foods high in refined carbohydrates has done much more harm than good to the whole world. What exactly happened, and what about the healthy Mediterranean diet?

Let's start with Keys' studies. First of all, the biologist, when selecting the famous seven countries, deliberately chose only those confirming his theories (many fats = many diseases; few fats = few diseases), discarding for instance countries such as Germany, France, Switzerland or Sweden, where the consumption of fats was high but the incidence of heart disease was not.

In addition, various methodological errors have emerged in his research: just to mention one, the surveys in the island of Crete were made during Lent, when the consumption of meat and cheese was much lower than normal. Most importantly, the study did not take into account the fact that, in the 1950s, food in southern Europe was heavily impoverished by the consequences of the Second World War, which had brought poverty and devastation everywhere; many typical local products (meat and dairy products, therefore fats) were not consumed as usual. Already during his years in Italy, Keys complained about how the outside world was contaminating the healthy local habits, with meat and dairy products that appeared in restaurants. He, however, did not evaluate

---

[12] AA.VV., *Seven Countries: A Multivariate Analysis of Death and Coronary Heart Disease*, Harvard University Press, 1980 ISBN 0674802373

[13] TIME Vol. 183, NO. 24 | 2014 di Bryan Walsh: "Ending the war on fat".

the possibility that the newfound well-being was simply making the real local eating habits emerge again[14].

Let's open a recipe book from 1935 and read what they say about the traditional cuisine of sunny Sardinia, one of the most beautiful islands in Italy[15]:

"One of the preferred ways to prepare short pasta is to cook it in lamb or pork fat... together with pieces of lamb or pork, diced tomatoes, chopped garlic and curd, all with a little water and salt and moistened with a little game broth, when there is". The gnocchi are "served with tomato or meat sauce and pecorino cheese". The polenta is accompanied by "minced salted pork, chunks of sausage and grated cheese".

The traditional Italian cuisine is full of fat, not only in the dressings (butter in the north, lard in the center, olive oil in the south), but also in the meats: pork, for instance, is consumed everywhere especially in the form of cured meats. Cheeses are the quintessence of the local culinary culture; eggs were, especially in the past, indispensable as a source of low-cost food... and what about ice cream, a great Italian tradition?

There are similar examples all around the world:

Jews living in Yemen (a diet rich in animal fats) have very different levels of diabetes and heart disease than Yemeni Jews living in Israel (a diet low in animal fats but rich in sugar)[16].

The Eskimos, who have a diet very rich in animal fats, are practically immune from the heart diseases, and usually very resistant, so much that they have been spoken of as "paradox of the Inuits"[17].

Okinawa, Japan, has the highest average life expectancy in the country, with very high consumption of pork and lard[18].

Delicious French cuisine is a triumph of saturated fat: butter, cheese, eggs, cream, meat and pate. Yet the incidence of coronary heart disease is among the lowest in Europe, and touches its lowest peaks precisely in those regions, such as Gascony, where goose and duck liver are considered like a religion[19].

---

[14] Wise Traditions in Food, Farming and the Healing Arts, *periodico della Weston A. Price Foundation, Primavera 2000*

[15] "Recipes of all nations", 1935, Marcelle Azra Hincks as Countess Morphy

[16] Case Studies in Physiology and Nutrition, Lynne Berdanier,Carolyn D. Berdanier, CRC Press, 2009

[17] Coronary heart disease in Greenland Inuit: a paradox. Implications for western diet patterns, Dyerberg J, Arctic Medical Research, 1989

[18] "Nourishing Traditions : The Cookbook that Challenges Politically Correct Nutrition and the Diet Dictocrats", Sally Fallon, Mary Enig, 2001

This information clearly contradicts popular beliefs about fats, which are still based on Keys' assumptions. Who is right? Let's start from biochemistry to get an answer.

A Matter of Curves

Fats, or lipids, are organic substances that are not soluble in water.

Most of the edible fats are composed of three molecules called fatty acids bonded together by a molecule called glycerol or glycerin (which is also found in many cosmetics, and which can also be used as a laxative). The resulting fat is called triglyceride.

The fatty acids that make up triglycerides can be classified as follows:

Saturated fatty acids have a molecular structure characterized by so-called single bonds, and for this reason their molecules are rigid and straight, and they compact thickly. This allows them to be solid at room temperature (e.g. butter).

In monounsaturated fatty acids, instead, the molecular chain has, at some point, a double bond, which causes it to make a "curve". This makes it more difficult for molecules to compact and, in fact, these fats are generally liquid at room temperature (think of olive oil).

Polyunsaturated fatty acids have two double bonds and therefore an even more complicated molecular structure, because of which they are liquid even when refrigerated and turn easily rancid. The most common are omega 3 and omega 6, also called essential fats because our body cannot produce them on its own[20].

---

[19] Ferrieres, J. (2004). "The French Paradox; Lessons for other countries". Heart 90 (1): 107–111.doi:10.1136/heart.90.1.107. PMC 1768013. PMID 14676260.

[20] Nelson, D. L.; Cox, M. M. (2000). Lehninger, Principles of Biochemistry (3rd ed.). New York: Worth Publishing. ISBN 1-57259-153-6.

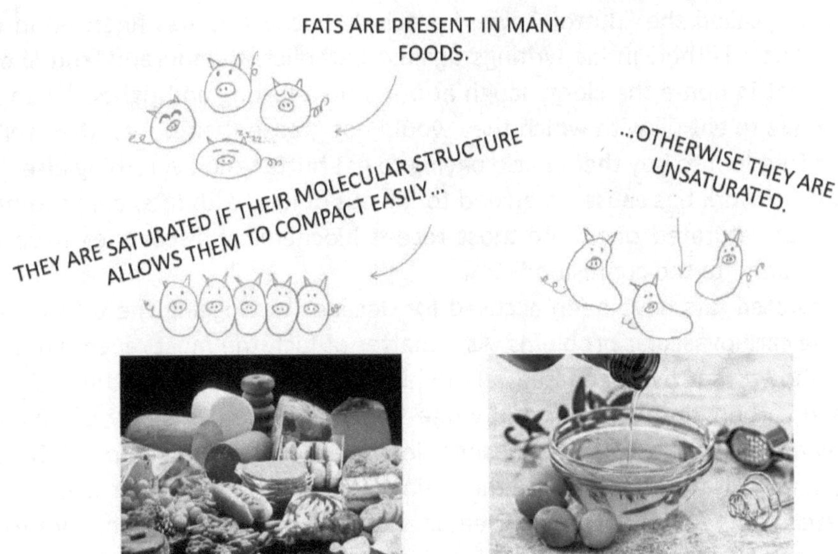

Foods generally contain a mix of the three types of fatty acids. Foods of animal origin (red meat, dairy products, etc.) contain about 40-60% of saturated fats, while plant-based ones (olive oil, dried fruit) contain a preponderance of monounsaturated and polyunsaturated acids. The only exceptions are fatty fishes (like salmons: of animal origin but rich in unsaturated fats) and tropical oils (palm, coconut: very saturated, despite their vegetable origin).

Having said that, what are the effects of these types of fats on our bodies? Opinions about who are the good guys and who are the bad guys have not always been in agreement over time. Let's try to understand something more.

The Butter Tower

In ancient times, animal fats, thanks to their power to provide reserve energy, were held in high esteem, especially in periods most subject to famine. Even in the Middle Ages, the wealthier classes of Northern Europe began to buy from the Church special indulgences that allowed them to consume this food even in prohibited periods, such as Lent, without upsetting the Creator. At a certain point, the trade in these special indulgences became a real affair for the Vatican, so much so that one of the towers of the cathedral of Rouen, in

France, is called the "Butter Tower" precisely because it was financed in this way. Martin Luther, in his writings against Catholics, thundered: "You should know that in Rome the clergy laugh at our stolen fasting and rights, forcing us foreigners to eat oil with which they would not grease their boots, then selling us the freedom to buy them back, paying to eat butter and everything else!"[21].

If Keys' work has caused mankind to fall out of love with fats, demonizing in particular saturated ones, the most recent biochemical discoveries have put some order into the confusion:

Saturated fats have been accused for decades of clogging the arteries and causing cardiovascular problems. As a matter of fact, the most recent studies[22] have shown that hydrogenated fats (which we will soon meet), the excess of refined carbohydrates (sugar and white flour), and the deficiency of minerals and vitamins (in particular magnesium, iodine, selenium and vitamin C, B6 and B12), and not saturated fats, are the main culprits of these problems.

Later in the book, we will see in detail the role of carbohydrates in cardiovascular problems; for now, we just need to note that the best way to treat heart disease is not to focus on reducing saturated fats, but to maintain a diet as balanced as possible and rich in nutrients, as well as poor in refined carbohydrates.

In addition, saturated fats have many beneficial effects on the body and are indeed essential for life itself: they play an essential role in fixing calcium to the bones; they protect the liver from toxins (including alcohol); they strengthen the immune system; they play an essential role in the production of hormones and in the proper functioning of nerve fibers. Eliminating them from the diet is, therefore, a terrible idea[23].

As far as monounsaturated fats are concerned, they have long been recognized as "good", and it is true: they protect the heart by reducing blood pressure; they lower the risk of heart disease and protect against inflammation[24]. Don't be afraid to dress your salad with plenty of extra virgin olive oil!

---

[21] "La mia vita al burro", Philippe Léveillé, 2015

[22] Added Sugar Intake and Cardiovascular Diseases Mortality Among US Adults. Quanhe Yang, PhD; Zefeng Zhang, MD, PhD; Edward W. Gregg, PhD; W. Dana Flanders, MD, ScD; Robert Merritt, MA; Frank B. Hu, MD, PhD, *JAMA Intern Med.* 2014;174(4):516-524. doi:10.1001/jamainternmed.2013.13563.

[23] Y MARY ENIG, PHD, IN THE MAGAZINE *Wise Traditions in Food, Farming and the Healing Arts*, Spring 2004.

[24] Egert S, Kratz M, Kannenberg F, Fobker M, Wahrburg U. "Effects of high-fat and low-fat diets rich in monounsaturated fatty acids on serum lipids, LDL size and indices of lipid peroxidation in

As for polyunsaturated fats, not all of them are so beneficial. For instance, omega 3 (abundant in fatty fish and dried fruit) fight inflammation, help control blood clotting and reduce blood pressure. Omega 6, however, (which most of us have no difficulty in taking, think that in the Western diet the ratio to omega 3 is 10 to 1!) can be harmful to the heart and, according to some studies[25], responsible, if consumed in too high quantities, even for damage to the liver and immune system, digestive disorders, depression and reduced growth. This is because, for the biochemical reasons seen above, these fats turn easily rancid. The process of rancidity involves a series of chemical transformations that generate, among other by-products, also some free radicals, real "wandering mines" in our body responsible for cellular damage and aging of tissues. These fats are present in some industrial vegetable oils, as well as in many snacks and packaged foods.

Zombie Fats

A very special class of fats that we have not yet mentioned deserves a separate mention: hydrogenated fats. They are the real bad guys. Worse than Cruella de Vil and Darth Vader put together. And this time there is no doubt. These are artificially modified fats, and therefore not present in nature. Hydrogenation adds hydrogen atoms to polyunsaturated fat molecules (normally the cheapest soy, corn, cotton and canola oils are used, often already rancid from the extraction process) to transform them artificially into fats that are solid instead of liquid. The advantage for producers is that they have a much cheaper food base than butter, and a very long shelf life. Margarine is made up of hydrogenated fats: place a pat of margarine on the kitchen table; it will remain unaltered for days, without being attacked by microorganisms, thanks to the partially hydrogenated fats.

What makes hydrogenated fats so lethal for us? The fact that, because of the hydrogenation process, it is very easy for fat molecules to undergo a

healthy non-obese men and women when consumed under controlled conditions". *Eur J Nutr.* 2011;50(1):71-79. PMID: 20521076 www.ncbi.nlm.nih.gov/pubmed/20521076.

[25] FOOD REVIEWS INTERNATIONAL Vol. 20, No. 1, pp. 77–90, 2004 Omega-6/Omega-3 Essential Fatty Acid Ratio and Chronic Diseases Artemis P. Simopoulos* The Center for Genetics, Nutrition and Health, Washington, D.C., USA

further chemical transformation that makes them trans fats, terrible toxins for our body. In fact, the enzymes that process fats do not recognize these "zombies" as such and are not able to process them. Their consumption is linked to atherosclerosis, coronary heart disease and, supposedly, risks of stroke, diabetes and obesity[26].

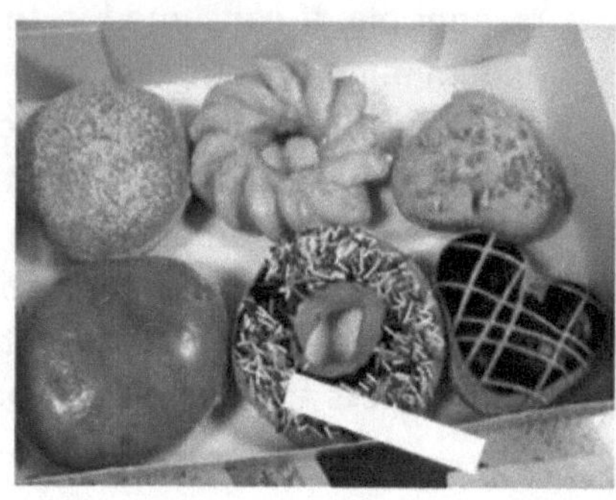

BEWARE OF HYDROGENATED FATS: THESE ARE ARTIFICIALLY CREATED FATS, WHICH HAVE DEVASTATING EFFECTS ON HEALTH !

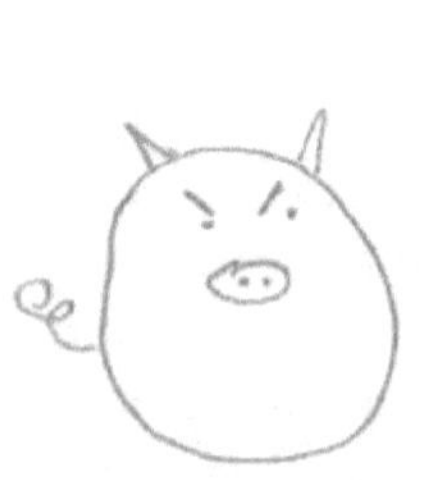

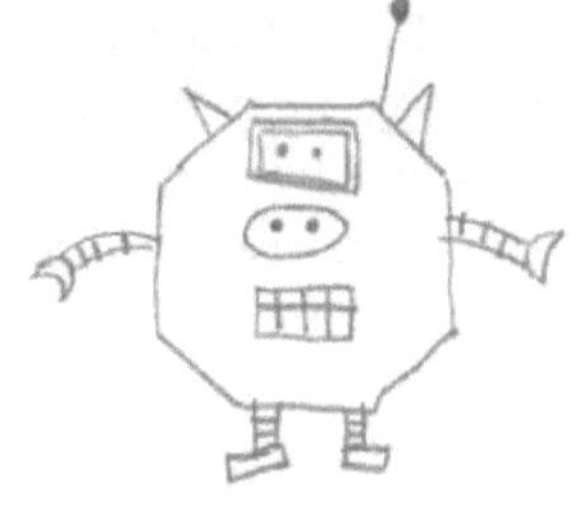

Besides margarine, hydrogenated fats are mainly contained in commercial products, including candies, chocolate bars, ice creams, bakery goods, frozen meals, TV dinners, salty snacks and fast food. Stay away from them! Don't hesitate to look for the words "hydrogenated" or "partially hydrogenated fats" on the labels. Pay attention also to the simple wording "vegetable fats" ... in reality, the best thing you can do is to avoid processed foods.

---

[26] Booyens J, Louwrens CC, Katzeff IE., The role of unnatural dietary trans and cis unsaturated fatty acids in the epidemiology of coronary artery disease., in Med Hypotheses., vol. 25, n° 3, 1988, p. 175–82,

To summarize: no fear of fats, not even saturated fats, if these are found in natural products. Mother Nature is not stupid and makes us find in unprocessed products substances that are good for us, in the right proportions. Balance saturated, polyunsaturated and monounsaturated fats by consuming many different foods: the ideal would be to distribute these three types of fats equally.

Moreover, within the polyunsaturated category, the ratio between omega 3 and 6 should also be one to one. As a guide, you can read Appendix C at the end of the book, which informs you about the content of the different types of fats in many foods.

A little fat will not hurt; of course, it cannot be the basis of the diet, especially for its high calorie content. We will return to the subject later, with a detailed look at the relationship between fat and body weight.

Stop eating processed foods, with their hydrogenated fats and with their dangerous disproportions of polyunsaturated fats.

4.Carbohydrates

"You sold your soul the day you put on that first pair of Jimmy Choo's! You don't deserve them, you eat carbs!"
Emily Charlton (Emily Blunt), The Devil Wears Prada

Over the last few years, carbohydrate has experienced a monstrous decline in popularity. Almost like a former disgraced star, it has gone from being the base of the famous food pyramid, source of energy, foundation of nutrition... to represent absolute evil, the main cause of weight gain and, in some cases, of even more serious problems.

Let's try to sort things out. Chemically speaking, carbohydrates are a family of molecules with some common characteristics, including the presence of atoms of carbon, oxygen and hydrogen organized in the form of a chain[27]. The simplest carbohydrates have a single link chain and are called monosaccharides or simple sugars. Some of the main monosaccharides are glucose (also called dextrose), the most common in nature; fructose (abundant in fruit) and galactose (present in milk).

Combine two monosaccharides and you will have a small chain made up of two rings: a disaccharide. The most known is saccharose (what we commonly call sugar), which is obtained by combining glucose and fructose; lactose (a molecule of glucose and one of galactose), which is the sugar of milk; maltose (two molecules of glucose) found in cereals.

As the chain lengthens, more complex and "long" carbohydrates are formed: polysaccharides. These include glycogen (which we will talk about later) and starch, which is contained in cereals, legumes and potatoes.

Gandhi and Sugar

In the thirties of the last century, an Indian mother was worried about her son's health. He seemed to be gobbling absurd doses of sugar every day, becoming a real addict of this substance. Since there was apparently no way to satisfy the hunger for sweetness, his mother grabbed the child and dragged

[27] *Long Island University* (May 29, 2013). "The Chemistry of Carbohydrates" (PDF). brooklyn.liu.edu.

him for miles under the scorching sun to reach her idol - none other than Mahatma Gandhi - and ask him for help.

Gandhi listened to the request, then waited in silence for a few moments, meditating, and finally told the mother to return after two weeks. Perplexed, the woman obeyed.

Fifteen days later, the scene was repeated. This time, Gandhi told the child that he should consume less sugar, and the little one promised he would do his best. The mother, however, was too curious, and could not help but ask the Master why he had waited two weeks.

"Two weeks ago," Gandhi replied, "I too had an obsession with sugar. I needed this time to get rid of it!"

From a spiritual point of view, the story teaches that great men want to support with the practice of their own lives the good advice they give; on the more concrete and practical side, it shows us, with a smile, how easy it is for everyone to indulge in sweet sugar.

Why, in general, do we love the sweet taste so much? Simply because we could not live without sugar.

Simple sugars are the gasoline of our organism. At every moment of our life, every cell of ours burns, inside tiny furnaces called mitochondria, glucose and oxygen to produce energy (we will see this process in detail). The energy we need to make the heart beat, to move, to breathe, to think... comes mainly from sugars. Our nervous system, in particular, is a glucose devourer; it needs more than a hundred grams a day, otherwise we can get to the loss of consciousness. However, you may be disoriented at this point. If that is the case, it would seem that in order to live it is necessary to continuously swallow sugar lumps. Luckily, that is not the case. Let us see why.

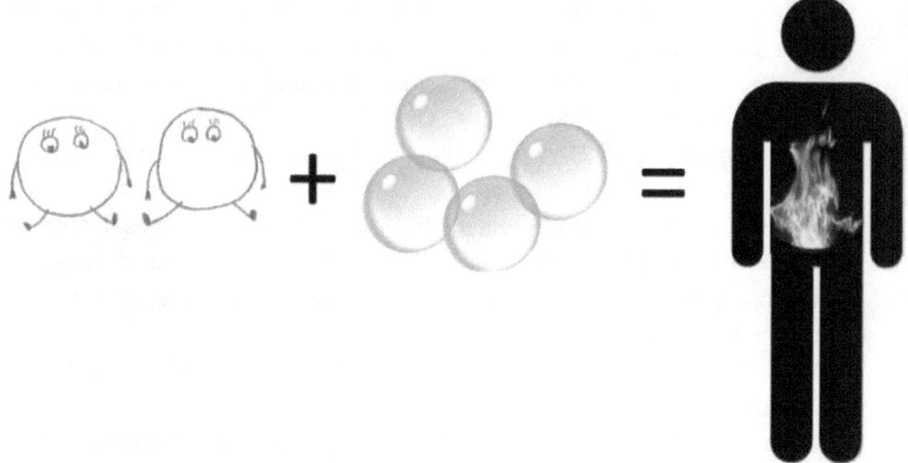

The Lament of the Pharaoh

Met an old friend whose name is Hatshepsut. She was born in Egypt more than three thousand five hundred years ago, and she was a female pharaoh. The voices about her seem to be very discordant: some portray her as a beautiful woman, pacifist and much loved by her people, while others saw her as a hag thirsty for power.

Regardless of the real personality of this nice fifty-year-old lady (this was her age when she died), we are interested here in her state of health. The fact is that, thanks to careful examinations made on the mummy, it emerged that Hatshepsut was obese, diabetic and full of tooth decay[28].

The same problems are quite common to most of the Egyptian mummies analyzed so far, along with heart disease and hypertension. The paradoxical fact is that the ancient Egyptians were certainly not a people who fed on fast food and gummy candies. On the contrary, the foods that prevailed in their

---

[28] *Tooth May Have Solved Mummy Mystery*, By JOHN NOBLE WILFORDJUNE 27, 2007, New York Times

diet would be applauded by most modern nutritionists: the fertile valleys of the Nile provided them with plenty of whole grains and fresh fruit and vegetables. Sugar was unknown; at most, they would sweeten a little with honey. And the consumption of meat, especially red meat, was reduced to a minimum (oxen were too precious; they were used to work the fields).

We already know that complex carbohydrates are nothing more than long chains of simple carbohydrates. Our digestive system just takes these chains in its hand and a little at a time breaks them into their basic rings. The lesson, which can be a bit shocking, is this: any carbohydrate is transformed by our body into simple sugars, such as fructose and glucose.

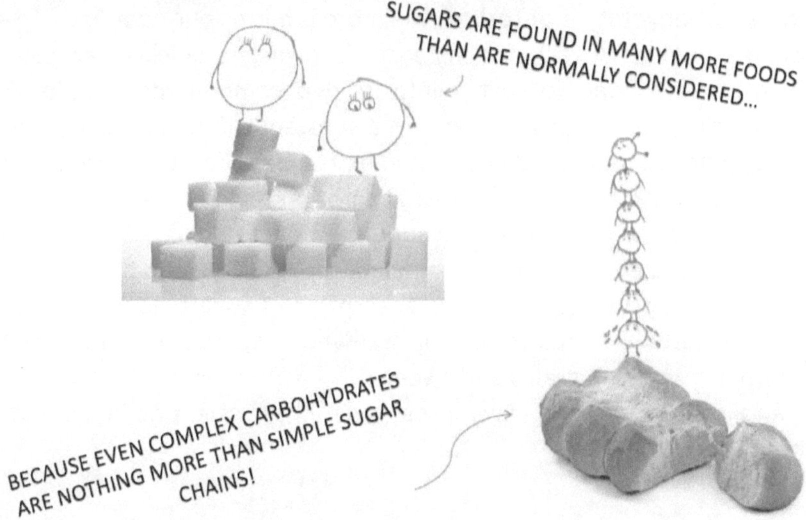

It doesn't matter if we swallow organic spelt or a chocolate: everything becomes simple sugars once inside us. Exactly like that: when you eat any type of cereal, even the healthiest, most wholemeal and organic, in the end what comes to your body is the same that would come if you ate spoonfuls of sugar from the pantry. And the same applies to all foods containing starch, which, as we have seen above, is a carbohydrate: bread, rice, pasta, potatoes, biscuits, and any cereal. That's why we don't have to consume sugar all the time to stay alive.

In addition, this explains the health problems of poor Hatshepsut (may she rest in peace) and her people: despite the fact that the foods they were eating were undoubtedly healthy and plant-based, the diet was highly unbalanced because it was based exclusively on carbohydrates and deprived, or greatly deficient, of the other essential nutrients that we have met so far, primarily proteins and fats. And any kind of unbalanced diet, as we believe is becoming evident, is lethal to our bodies. Obesity, diabetes and heart disease are some of the problems associated with diets that are too rich in carbohydrates.

Be careful, however: the source of carbohydrates is not indifferent: it is not a good idea to replace the wholemeal bread you eat at meals with chocolate bars. While it is true that all carbohydrates become simple sugars, it should be stressed that the effect that a carbohydrate has on our body depends mainly on its ability to be absorbed and metabolized more or less slowly. In general, the faster a carbohydrate is absorbed, the more it harms our body[29].

Saccharose (white sugar), for instance, is digested quickly because it is enough to break a bond to split it into its two components: simple sugars glucose and fructose. For this reason, it is a substance that is basically harmful to our body, and it should be consumed in extreme moderation. Starches have more chains to break, but to make their absorption really "slow" it is necessary to take them from whole grains, because the fibers contained in them slow down digestion and absorption. The same goes for fruit sugars: the presence of fibers and other substances makes the absorption of sugars slower. Therefore, in fact, taking carbohydrates from fruit and whole grains is much better than taking them from refined grains and sweets.

In the following chapters, we will see in detail the scientific demonstration of all these concepts.

5. Let's Take a First Stock of the Situation

"One cannot think well, love well, sleep well, if one has not dined well"
Virginia Wolf

---

[29] Am J Clin Nutr. 2007 Mar;85(3):724-34. Effects of a reduced-glycemic-load diet on body weight, body composition, and cardiovascular disease risk markers in overweight and obese adults, Maki KC, Rains TM, Kaden VN, Raneri KR, Davidson MH.

So far, we have met the molecules protagonists of our inner biochemistry and we are only at the beginning of the journey; however, by putting together the general information we have seen so far, there are already some themes that can make us think, before we even discuss metabolism and explore the effects of nutrition on health and body weight.

Just like in a thriller, we seek clues and points in common between the stories we have told so far. Before you continue reading, try to scroll briefly through the previous pages; can you see them?

There are at least two of them.

First, the importance of variety. We have seen that there are substances that our body cannot produce, and which must necessarily be taken from the outside: essential amino acids, omega three, omega six, vitamins, and minerals. We have also seen how diverse and varied the foods that contain them are. Moreover, we believe it is very clear from the previous paragraphs that no fundamental nutrient can be left behind: all of them are indispensable to our lives.

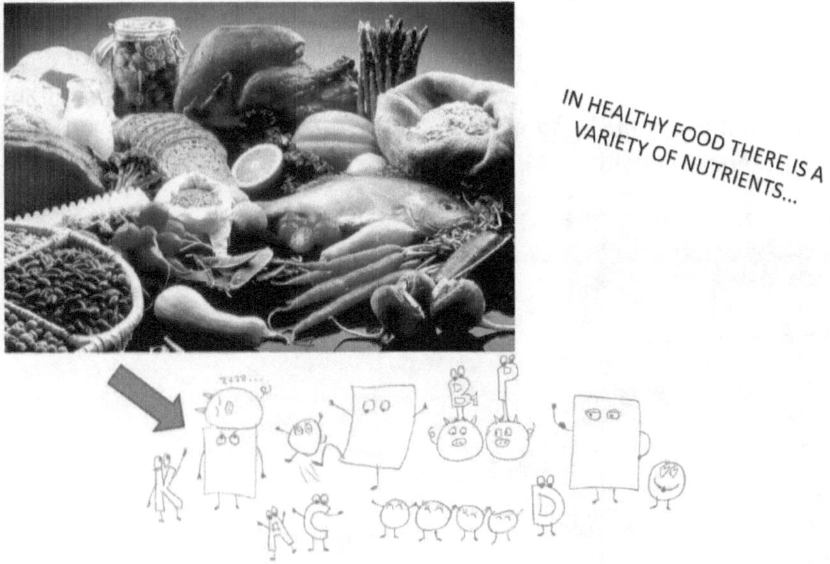

Therefore, first, diets that exclude a type of nutrient are actually harmful; moreover, within one's own diet, the more varied the foods, the more benefits one has. These may sound like "grandma's" statements, trivial and obvious, but how many of us really pay attention to them? If you always eat the same things, in the long run this will deprive your body of something essential. Give yourself the mission to experiment and vary; the benefit will be enormous.

The second point is the most important. Perhaps, it is the most fundamental advice of the whole book. Moving too far away from Mother Nature is detrimental. We have seen this, for instance, regarding soil impoverishment, trans fats, and carbohydrates from refined cereals.

Our digestive system and our metabolism have evolved over the millennia, "calibrating" on those simple foods that our ancestors have had as their only form of nourishment: fruit, vegetables, whole grains, meat, fish, dairy products, eggs, etc. Each industrial transformation of these foods adds, removes or modifies substances taking our body aback and leaving it in danger. So, just to mention two examples:

Don't fear the fat of a nice steak: it has a good proportion of saturated and monounsaturated fats, vital for us, and is accompanied by the proteins and other nutrients of the meat. Instead, fear the hydrogenated fat or omega 6 of that fast-food hamburger.

Don't fear the sugars of fresh fruit: the presence of fibers regulates their absorption, and vitamins and minerals counterbalance their presence. Instead, fear the sugar from the candy bars or sweets bought at the supermarket, or the sugar that (hush-hush) abounds in the fruit juice that you keep in the fridge and that seems so healthy.

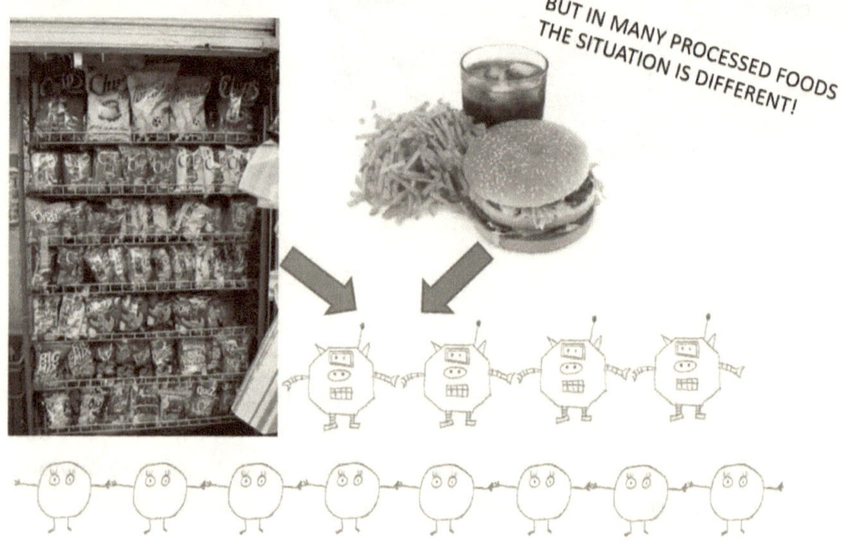

Remember: the closer it is to the way it is in nature, the better. Want to do a little experiment? Try for a month to feed yourself only with products that are identical, or very close to how they are found in nature, that is:

- grilled meat and fish
- fresh milk, unsweetened yogurt, homemade cheese and butter
- fresh fruit and vegetables
- whole grains (not industrial products containing whole grains ... we mean the actual grains: buckwheat, spelt, barley, brown rice...)
- fresh eggs
- extra virgin olive oil as a condiment

No sugar (meaning saccharose, now we know what it is!) and products that contain it; no non-wholegrain cereals and their derivatives (all that is done with white flour); no cured meat; no processed/industrial product at all.

At the end of the month, you may have some pleasant surprises; you may find yourself a few kilos lighter, even though you have not made any apparent sacrifice; you may also find yourself with more energy, more beautiful and healthier.

You have simply eaten things made to be eaten by you. This, however, is merely the beginning...

PART TWO

Metabolism

6. Enzymes and Hormones

There are two types of substances you need to familiarize with before we can talk about metabolism: enzymes and hormones.

The Man with a Hole in His Stomach

On June 6, 1822, William Beaumont, a doctor from a remote village on the island of Mackinac, Michigan, was alarmed by a loud gunshot coming from a nearby warehouse. He rushed to see what had happened, and to his enormous horror he found a guy in his twenties in a pool of blood. "A horrible wound", recounted the doctor in his memoirs, "the size of the palm of a hand. From the singed shirt were coming out pieces of ribs, cartilages and fragments of breakfast food. When the boy coughed, it was clear where they were coming from: the explosion had pierced his stomach." The poor guy, his name was Alexis St. Martin, had just accidentally fired a shot from his rifle.

Beaumont not only treated the boy's wound saving his life, but decided to have him live in his home (Alexis was poor and illiterate) giving him a job as an assistant. Why am I telling you this tear-jerking story? The reason is that Alexis' clinical case became unique in the history of medicine: when the wound healed, in the young man's body remained a sort of "window" open on his stomach, covered by a strip of skin. It was therefore possible to observe the digestive processes of poor William in real time.

Until then, the digestion of food was considered as a mechanical process of the bowels, which ground the ingested mouthfuls, at the most finished by an unspecified "fermentation".

What Beaumont, on the other hand, managed to observe by extracting a piece of meat from the "window" on the stomach, was that some foods melted little by little, turning into something else, probably because of some chemical substance.

Keeping Alexis at bay (he was rather hot-tempered and sometimes didn't appreciate too much the intrusions inside his body), Beaumont continued to observe, noting that in his tummy there was an acid liquid that had never been ingested by the boy, and deduced that it must have been produced by his stomach. He picked it out with a straw and observed how that juice digested several elements, which he closed in small vials. He noticed that the milk coagulated as soon as it arrived in the stomach, and that it took much less time to destroy the meat than the vegetables[30].

It is thanks to this curious doctor with no sense of privacy that the discovery of human digestive processes began. The mysterious juices that "melted" food, and that Beaumont closed in the tubes, work thanks to enzymes, the real protagonists of all digestion.

Enzymes are substances (primarily proteins) specialized in triggering chemical reactions in the body. They work like skilled workers: welders (joining two different molecules together to form a larger one) or shearers (dividing large molecules into smaller parts). The enzymes involved in the digestion of food belong to this second type.

---

[30] Harré, R. (1981). *Great Scientific Experiments*. Phaidon (Oxford). pp. 39–47. ISBN 0-7148-2096-2.

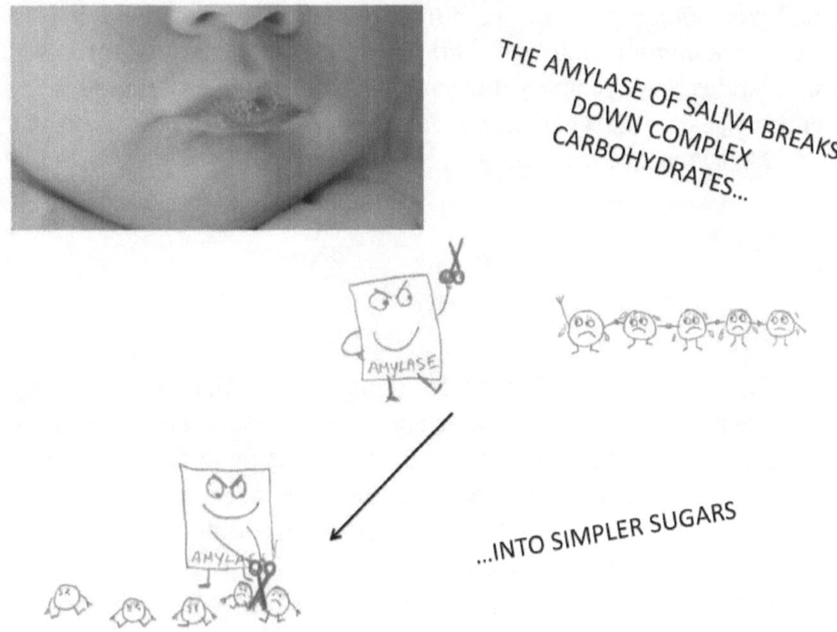

To better understand what we mean: remember, when we talked about proteins and amino acids, the example of the old inventor who scraps the materials of the landfill and then recomposes them? Well, the actions of this old man are carried out in our bodies by two types of enzymes: those that at first divide complex substances into simpler substances (such as proteins in amino acids) and those that then assemble simple substances into complex substances (from amino acids back to proteins).

We'll help you find some enzymes in your home. Don't worry, this doesn't mean you have to drill holes in your stomach. First, take a look at the label of the laundry detergent you have in the bathroom. Good chances are that in the composition of the product you'll find some name that ends in "ase" (such as Protease, Amylase or Lipase); "ase" is in fact the suffix that, in chemistry, identifies enzymes. In detergents, enzymes have recently been added more and more, precisely because of their ability to break down molecules of organic dirt (such as grease) into simpler substances that are easier to detach from the tissues.

Do you want another one? Put a finger in your mouth and take it out: your saliva contains two powerful enzymes: amylase and lipase. Both serve the purpose of starting to "break" the long chains of polysaccharides into simpler sugars. If you keep a piece of bread in your mouth and moisten it with saliva, after about a minute you will start to notice a vaguely sweet taste: the polysaccharides are becoming disaccharides, which the taste buds recognize. Our entire digestive system is studded with enzymes which play, as we will see, a key role in all metabolic processes.

Two Very Strange Villages

In the village of Salinas, Dominican Republic, something happens regularly that may appear on the verge of science fiction. Many girls (almost one in every hundred) turn into boys at the beginning of puberty, developing male sexual organs around the age of twelve. This experience is so normal that the Dominican Republic has created a third gender specifically for them, "pseudo-hermaphrodite" or, in the common language, "guevedoces"[31].

Interviewed by the BBC, 24-year-old Johnny says that he was born a girl, with the name of Felicita, and remained so until his transformation, which occurred spontaneously at the age of twelve. "When I was born, my parents and the doctors thought I was a girl, they would dress me in skirts and give me girls' toys, but I didn't really feel comfortable", explains Felicita-Johnny. "When I changed, I became happy with my life".

Let's now move southwest to Ecuador, from the Caribbean Sea to the cold Andes. In 1987, the South American doctor Jaime Guevara-Aguirre embarked on an adventurous holiday on horseback in this area, venturing out of the usual tourist routes. He arrived in a remote village where he met a group of people, all suffering from dwarfism: most of them did not reach more than one meter and ten in height. Intrigued by the fact, he decided to study the phenomenon. Almost ten years later, when data collection was enough, Jaime announced to the skeptical international scientific community that the strange people of the Andes were immune to one of the most devastating diseases of the contemporary world: cancer. Twenty-four years after the discovery, there was still no case of cancer among the dwarfs of the Andes, against 17% of the local population of normal stature[32].

---

[31] "Sembrano bambine ma a 12 anni diventano maschi", GIACOMO TALIGNANI, from the italian newspaper "Repubblica", 29th of September 2015

What do these two weird stories have in common? In both cases, hormones change the rules of the game.

We can think of hormones as a sort of "keys" that activate specific "locks" in our cells. They are produced by different glands (e.g. pancreas, glands over the kidneys, thyroid, testicles and ovaries) precisely to enable the activation or deactivation of certain biochemical processes. They are interesting for us because the metabolism of the human body is made up of numerous processes which, in fact, are "opened" or "closed" by these precious keys. To better understand, let's quickly look, as an example, at what happens in the two amazing villages we have just described.

Regarding the strange transformations of Salinas, the population is affected by a rare genetic syndrome that delays the action of a hormone called dihydrotestosterone. All fetuses in the womb have a protrusion called tubercle between the legs; at eight weeks, dihydrotestosterone activates some receptors of the tubercle that turn it into a penis (this, of course, only if the sex is male: for females the process leads to the formation of the clitoris). In Salinas, this hormone begins to be produced only with puberty, and for this reason the penis develops only at this time.

Even for the people in the Andes, the cause of the phenomenon is to be found in a genetic syndrome (Laron's syndrome): Here, the "locks" that get opened by a hormone called somatropin (or growth hormone, GH) are missing. Under normal conditions, GH basically causes more amino acids to enter the cells, increasing protein synthesis, and thus growth. This explains the dwarfism: without receptors, this process is blocked. But what about resistance to cancer?

---

[32] Elena Meli, "Il villaggio dove non esistono tumori né il diabete", from the italian newspaper "Corriere della Sera", 3rd of March 2011

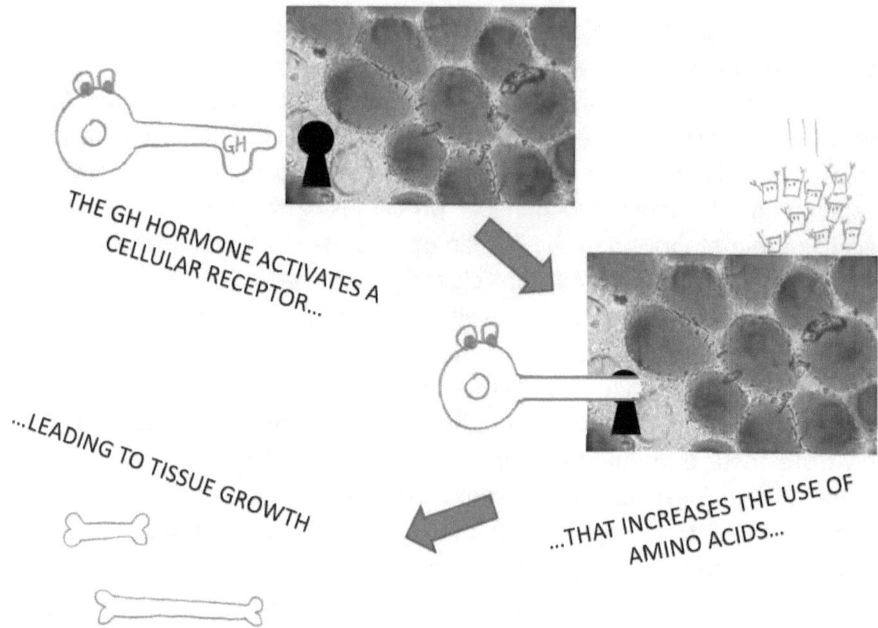

A tumor is caused by cells "gone haywire" which reproduce without control; the lack of GH receptors causes a significant reduction in the trigger for cancer formation. It is therefore no surprise that cancer researchers are looking at this hormone with a special focus.

7. The Metabolism of Carbohydrates

"With devotion's visage, and pious action we do sugar o'er the devil himself."
William Shakespeare

The Most Unfortunate Marathon Runner in History

One of the most curious stories of all the modern Olympics is that of the Japanese marathon runner Shizo Kanakuri. The athlete was among the favorites in the races of 1912, in Sweden. Shizo was maintaining an excellent race pace and had steadily positioned himself in the lead of the marathon. At the 30th kilometer, however, something happened. Suffering from an increasing drop in energy, the fast Japanese was tempted by the offer of a spectator who was watching the race from his own garden and drank a glass of raspberry juice. In addition, due to the heat, Shizo accepted the invitation to rest for a few minutes, in the cool, inside the house of the man. Here, he fell into deep sleep, waking up only when the race had already been over for several hours; he had been reported missing and the police were looking for him everywhere.

Out of shame, Shizo disappeared and returned home with makeshift means. In 1962, a Swedish journalist found him in Japan, and in 1967, by then 67 years old, he was invited to Stockholm to finish his legendary marathon, on the occasion of the 55th anniversary of the Olympic Games. He resumed the marathon with great sportiness right from the house where he had fallen asleep, and ended it with a time of 54 years, 8 months, 6 days, 5 hours, 32 minutes, 20 seconds and 3 tenths, the longest in history[33].

Shizo's strange story reveals a detail that the readers who are passionate about this sport will not have missed: it is not by chance that the small crisis

---

[33] "The Olympics' Strangest Moments: Extraordinary But True Tales from the History of the Olympic Games", Geoff Tibballs, Pavilion Books, 2008

that caused it all happened just at the 30th kilometer (approximately the 18th mile). Marathon runners know well the feeling that gets you, more or less, at this point of the marathon: the race suddenly becomes much more difficult, and a growing physical discomfort rises in the body. The feeling is so widespread that it has a name: bonking, bumping into a "wall". What happens exactly at the 30th kilometer?

As always, we let this question be the starting point for understanding something more about the biochemistry of our bodies; in detail, about how we produce and use energy. It is easy to imagine that the subject is therefore the metabolism of carbohydrates, which we know to be the primary source of energy of the body.

Now that we have the tools to better understand what our body does with each substance that makes up food, we start by following what happens to a piece of bread after we put it in the mouth.

We have already seen that the digestion of carbohydrates begins right here: the enzyme amylase starts to break the bonds of the long chains of starch, disassociating them. Since the food does not stay in the mouth long, many times this process does not have time to be completed, so the amylase appears again in the digestive process: after leaving the stomach (in which the carbohydrates do not undergo major changes), our piece of bread (now all mangled) is in fact sprayed with juices produced by the pancreas, in which we find the same enzyme. Its job can therefore be completed: the starch chains have been broken; the starch polysaccharide has been transformed into many disaccharides; each of them is called maltose[34].

There is still one bond left to break; another enzyme, this time produced by the walls of the small intestine, takes care of it: the maltase, which breaks down every molecule of maltose into two molecules of glucose.

The intestine also produces two other enzymes specifically for the other two disaccharides (do you remember them?): sucrase breaks saccharose into fructose and glucose, and lactase breaks lactose into glucose and galactose.

At this point, the simple sugars are absorbed by the walls of the small intestine (the famous villi), through which they enter the bloodstream. Fructose and galactose are mostly converted into glucose as soon as they pass

---

[34] January 1970Volume 58, Issue 1, Pages 96–107, "Carbohydrate Digestion and Absorption", Gary M. Gray, M.D., Department of Medicine, Stanford University School of Medicine, Stanford, California

through the liver, which is why about 95% of the monosaccharides in the blood are glucose.

Now to the simplest case: the one where glucose thus entered into the bloodstream is used directly by a cell. Let's take the case, for instance, of a glucose molecule that reaches a neuron (one of the cells that compose our brain).

First, glucose must pass through the cell wall to enter it. A protein, called Glut, takes care of it. Do you know those insistent "tourist-catchers", that in the holiday resorts try to haul tourists in the street to get them into their restaurant? Well, Glut does, more or less, the same.[35]

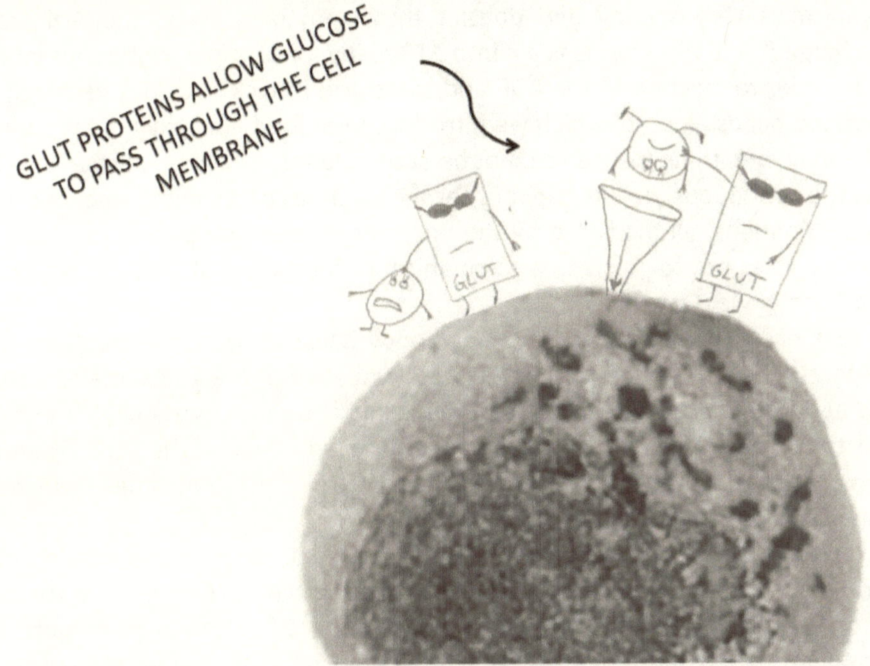

Once the cell has seized glucose, what does it do with it? If you remember, we have seen that the ultimate goal of sugars is to produce the energy that keeps us alive and that allows us to move, think, breathe, digest... Our body is composed of something like 100.000.000.000.000 (one hundred thousand

---

[35] Mol Aspects Med. Author manuscript; available in PMC 2014 Jul 21., Published in final edited form as: Mol Aspects Med. 2013 Apr-Jun; 34(0): 121–138. doi: 10.1016/j.mam.2012.07.001 PMCID: PMC4104978 NIHMSID: NIHMS394095; The SLC2 (GLUT) Family of Membrane Transporters; Mike Mueckler and Bernard Thorens

billion!) cells, and each of them, at any time, needs to be able to live and function.

To perform all these processes, our body uses a substance called ATP (adenosine triphosphate). We can imagine every molecule of ATP as a small, charged battery. ATP is used for every process that consumes energy: for instance, the contraction of muscles, the passage of impulses in the nerves, the multiplication of cells to grow or replace damaged ones, the functioning of enzymes.... Without ATP, we would stop immediately[36].

Once an ATP molecule has been used, it turns into ADP (adenosine diphosphate). ADP is nothing more than the "exhausted" version of ATP. Our organism is very sparing and doesn't throw anything away: the ADP gets "recharged" and transforms again into ATP ready for use, in a continuous cycle.

In order to "recharge" the ADP and transform it back into ATP, each cell in our body needs glucose, which we introduce with food, and oxygen, which we take while breathing (oxygen cannot be accumulated...which is why we have to breathe continuously). This happens through a series of chemical reactions and transformations, all mediated by the enzymes. We will simplify it as much as possible so as not to go crazy with chemical formulas, but still trying to have a clear idea of what goes on.

First of all, within every cell of our body, glucose must be "treated", i.e. prepared to be "burned" with oxygen. Still unaware of the gruesome fate that it is about to walk into, each glucose molecule is treated by specific enzymes, and transformed into a substance called pyruvate. Pyruvate is very different from sweet glucose: it is a yellowish acid with a pungent smell, which is sometimes used in cosmetics as a scrub.

This reaction alone produces energy: only by being transformed into pyruvate with this "treatment" by the enzymes, glucose, reacting with various other substances, can recharge four exhausted ADPs. However, it must be considered that the enzymes which treated glucose consumed energy, discharging two ATPs. Therefore, in the end, the balance of this first phase (called glycolysis) is two molecules of ATP. A bit thin for the needs of the cells, which is why the reactions must continue.[37]

---

[36] Knowles, J. R. (1980). "Enzyme-catalyzed phosphoryl transfer reactions". Annu. Rev. Biochem. 49: 877 919. PMID 6250450. doi:10.1146/annurev.bi.49.070180.004305

[37] Campbell, Neil A.; Williamson, Brad; Heyden, Robin J. (2006). Biology: Exploring Life. Boston, MA: Pearson Prentice Hall. ISBN 0-13-250882-6.

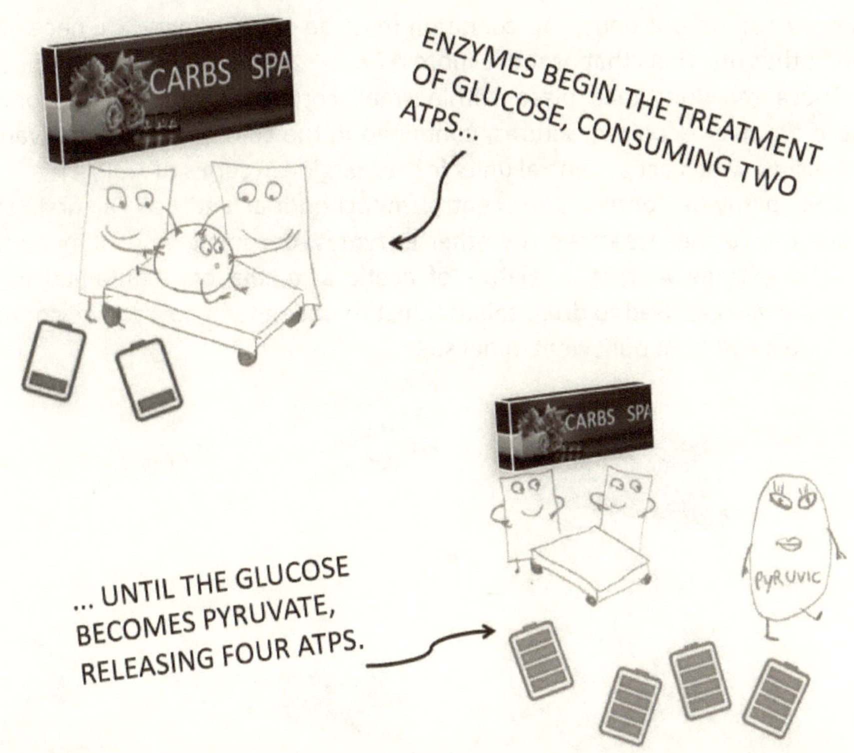

However, it is worth revealing a curiosity first: in more primitive organisms, such as yeasts, glycolysis is the only way to produce energy. For this reason, these organisms do not need oxygen, but only glucose. We are talking about yeasts that are used in the kitchen: in fact, the pyruvate, no longer used in successive phases, is transformed into carbon dioxide and ethanol.

Carbon dioxide is the gas that makes the dough rise, thus allowing cakes and bread to become soft and fluffy. We now know that this reaction starts from the glucose contained in the dough. As far as ethanol is concerned, this links us to another (very popular) use of yeasts: alcoholic fermentation. Even yeasts that transform grapes into wine or barley malt into beer use glycolysis starting from the glucose contained in these substances: ethanol is nothing but alcohol. The next time you enjoy a beer, you will know that all the credit belongs to glycolysis.

Under special circumstances (such as very intense physical exercise), we can also stop at this first stage of the process. However, given the enormous energy needs of our body, this condition must be extraordinary: we necessarily need other reactions that produce more ATP.

These reactions take place within small corpuscles called mitochondria. These are microscopic structures, contained in the cells of the most advanced organisms, which act as central units for recharging in series of ADP/ATPs.

The pyruvate enters the central/mitochondria and, as a first step, undergoes further treatment by other enzymes, becoming a substance called acetyl-coenzyme A. It is a relative of acetic acid, the one contained in the common vinegar used to dress salads... just to understand how far we continue to move away from our sweet initial sugar.

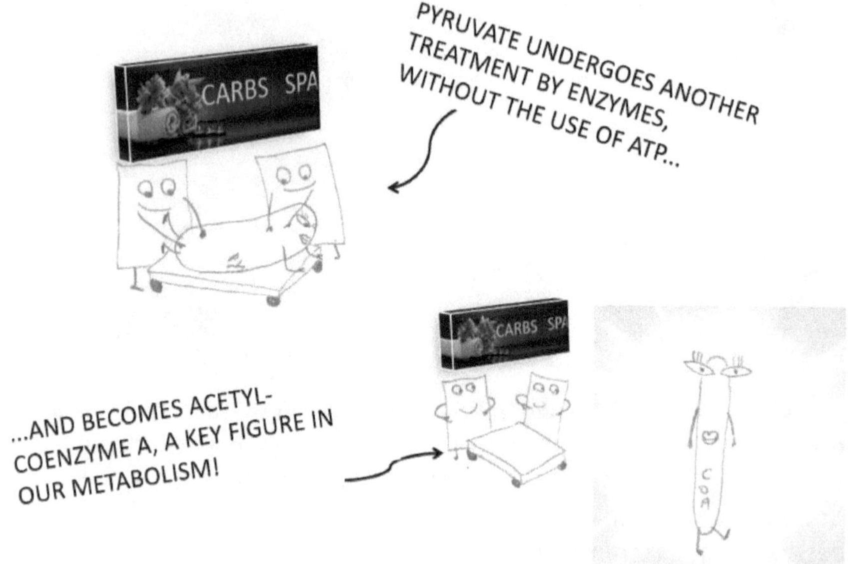

Here, we are at the heart of the process: acetyl-coenzyme A is ready to be "burned" by reacting with oxygen. "Burning" is clearly an improper term that only serves to give us an idea: what happens in the mitochondria is actually a series of reactions (mediated, needless to say, by enzymes) that, starting from acetyl-coenzyme A and oxygen, release the energy needed to recharge 36 ATPs for each original molecule of glucose used. It is therefore clear that the energy yield of this process is much greater than the minimum energy yield of glycolysis.

The set of reactions taking place in the mitochondria is called, in scientific terms, the Krebs cycle[38]. In addition to the ATP charged with energy for our lives, it produces various waste substances, including water and carbon dioxide. Every time we breathe, we throw out of the body with our own breath the carbon dioxide produced by billions of Krebs cycles into the mitochondria of our cells.

However, glucose that enters the cells is not always intended for immediate energy production. Sometimes, for instance after meals, there is more glucose in the bloodstream than what is needed. Our body, which is very foresighted, certainly does not throw it away, but stores it for lean times. Otherwise, we would be forced to eat all the time, just as we breathe all the time, and it would be a rather uncomfortable life. Instead, by storing excess glucose, we can use it later. For instance, the energy that makes you breathe at night, when you don't eat and there is little glucose in your blood, is released from the supplies accumulated after the meals of the day, when the glucose in circulation was abundant.

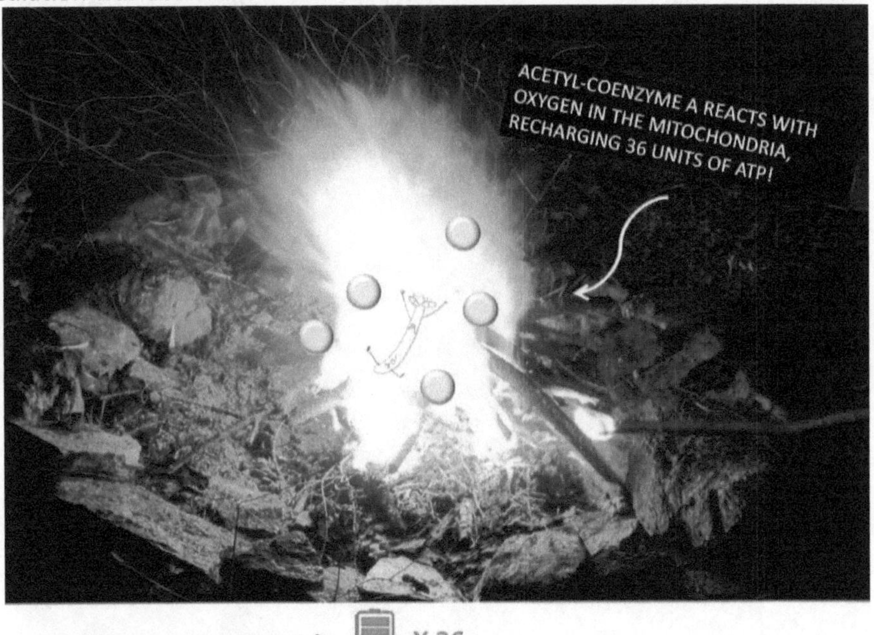

How does this reserve mechanism work? The cells responsible for this are mainly those of the muscles and liver. The glucose, once entered in these cells

[38] Lowenstein JM (1969). *Methods in Enzymology, Volume 13: Citric Acid Cycle*. Boston: Academic Press. ISBN 0-12-181870-5

thanks to the "tourist-catcher" Glut, gets stored if it is not immediately used for glycolysis and Krebs cycle.

To store glucose molecules, some enzymes in muscle and liver cells bind them to each other to form a polysaccharide called a glycogen. The glycogen is, therefore, nothing more than a stock of glucose in our body. About two thirds of the body's glycogen is stored in the muscles; the remaining third in the liver. When the body has to use these stocks, it simply "detaches" the glucose molecules from the glycogen one by one to use them; this task is carried out by the enzyme phosphorylase[39].

There is a limit to the glycogen that our body can store. Why is that? As we have already noticed, Mother Nature is not stupid. Glycogen, because of its structure, is a bit like a sponge, and every gram of glycogen binds about three grams of water to itself. Besides a certain amount, the space occupied would be really too much (unless we become walking aquariums); this is why there is a physiological limit to the amount of glycogen that can be stored in our bodies. This quantity varies according to many parameters; more or less, from about 350 to about 500 grams, in an adult organism (therefore, not that much).

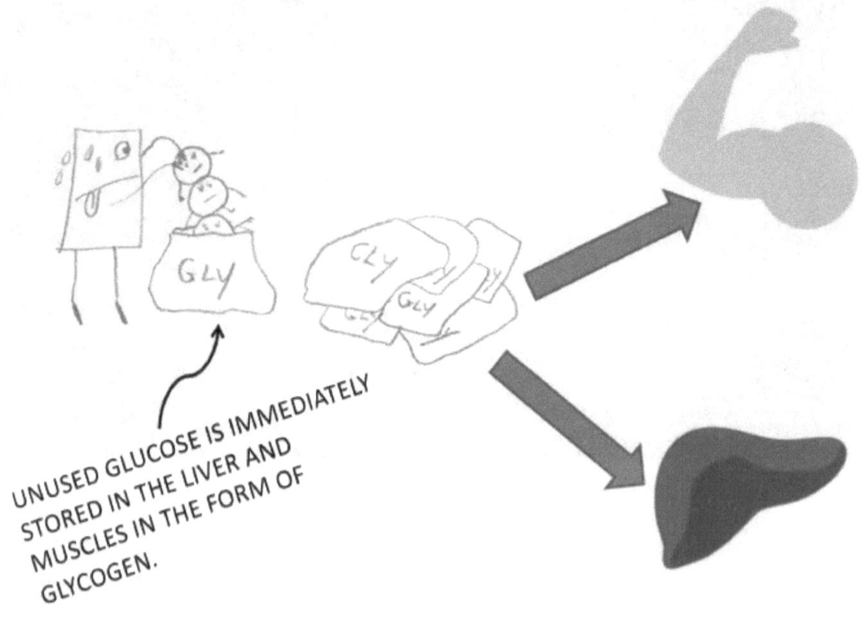

---

[39] Lodish; et al. (2007). *Molecular Cell Biology* (6th ed.). W. H. Freeman and Company. p. 658. ISBN 1429203145.

Once this space is used up, our body needs to transform sugars into something that can be stored in less space and more efficiently.

Well, yes, the brilliant solution of Mother Nature is to convert sugars into fat. The cells that can perform this unfortunate alchemy are those of the liver and those of adipose tissue.

When the glycogen stock is full, these cells give their mitochondria a counter-order: acetyl-coenzyme A molecules no longer need to be reacted with oxygen in the Krebs cycle; instead, they need to be kicked out of the mitochondria.

After that, various enzymes activate a series of reactions that ultimately result in the transformation of acetyl-coenzyme A into palmitic acid. Palmitic acid (so called because it was first discovered in palm oil) is a fatty acid. If you remember, fatty acids, when combined with glycerin (or glycerol) form triglycerides, the most common type of fat in our body.

Our liver, therefore, by combining fatty acids (palmitic acid) and glycerol, forms a triglyceride. Human flab, in other words, consists of molecules and molecules of triglycerides. The triglycerides coming out of the liver are guided to the adipose tissue, and there they accumulate to the delight of our dietician.

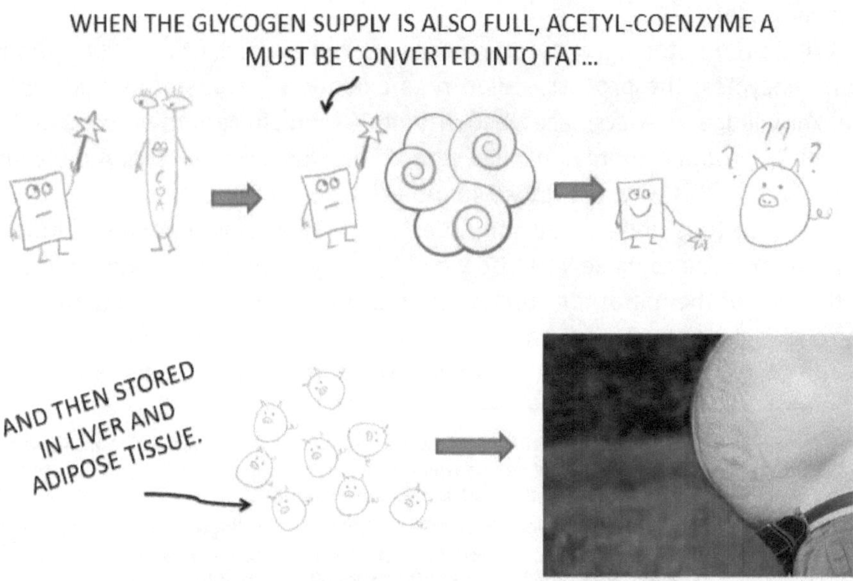

Adipose tissue is formed by cells specialized in the accumulation of fat. Each of us has between 10 and 30 billion of them, scattered throughout the body. Besides serving as a fat store, this tissue has a major function: it occupies the interstices, covers nerves, blood vessels and muscles, and acts as a protective buffer for various organs. It also isolates us from the cold[40].

A curiosity: a skinny person has the same number of fat cells as an obese person: in fact, by slimming and fattening, fat cells are not lost or gained, they are simply filled or emptied of fat. We could say that our billions of fat cells are slimming and fattening together with us. However, in the same way as it has been accumulated, the fat can be used. What would otherwise be the point of storing?

Muscle cells will first use blood glucose to produce the ATP needed for their function. When that is finished, they move on to the glycogen reserves of the muscles and liver: as we have seen above, the enzyme phosphorylase detaches the glucose molecules from it. But if the glycogen also finishes, the body must affect the fat reserves of the adipose tissue. The enzyme lipase, the number one enemy of fat reserves, takes care of this.

Lipase breaks down the triglycerides of fat cells into their original components: one molecule of glycerol and three of fatty acids. The whole thing enters the bloodstream, and the hungry cells plunder, in deficiency of their beloved sugar.

Within the mitochondria, fatty acids undergo a series of transformations by some enzymes; the process, called beta-oxidation[41], transforms them into an old knowledge of ours: acetyl-coenzyme A, which can then be used with oxygen to produce energy, just like when it derives from glucose. A molecule of fatty acids, in this way, provides 146 molecules of ATP.

We have thus understood the detail of the reactions that cause prolonged physical exercise to make you lose weight. But we have also solved the mystery of the wall of the marathon runner and the curse of the 30th kilometer of poor Shizo: the glycogen stored, on average, in a human body, is in fact enough only to run to that distance. The sense of exhaustion that appears is due to the

---

[40] *Stock, M. J.; Cinti, S. (2003). "Adipose Tissue / Structure and Function of Brown Adipose Tissue". Encyclopedia of Food Sciences and Nutrition.*
p. 29. ISBN 9780122270550. doi:10.1016/B0-12-227055-X/00008-0.

[41] Houten, Sander Michel; Wanders, Ronald J. A. (2010-03-02). "A general introduction to the biochemistry of mitochondrial fatty acid β-oxidation". *Journal of Inherited Metabolic Disease.* 33 (5): 469–477. ISSN 0141 8955. PMC 2950079. PMID 20195903. doi:10.1007/s10545-010-9061-2.

transition that the body must make from the consumption of glycogen to the consumption of fat; it is not by chance that the most advanced methods of training for this sport include techniques whose purpose should be to burn fat and glycogen at the same time.

A very brief summary before moving on, just to make sure we have a clear idea: All the carbohydrates we eat become simple sugars, mainly glucose. Glucose is used by our body's cells to produce energy (ATP). When there is more than what is needed, it is first accumulated in the liver and muscles in the form of glycogen. When the "space" available for glycogen is full, glucose becomes fat and enriches adipose tissue. On the contrary, if we need more glucose than the one available, we use the glycogen stock, transforming it back into glucose, and then the fat stock, transforming it straight into energy.

8. The Metabolism of Fats

"Is it better to be the lover or the loved one? Neither, if your cholesterol is over six hundred."
Woody Allen

A Paradoxical Fondue

For the French cheese fondue, you will need 17.6 ounces of Emmental, 17.6 ounces of Comté, 7.1 ounces of Beaufort (if you don't know these cheeses, I strongly recommend you taste them; you have no idea what you are missing...), a clove of garlic, a pinch of pepper, a tablespoon of starch and a couple of glasses of dry white wine.

Preparing it is easy: peel the garlic and rub it in a pot; pour the wine and bring to a boil, then add the cheese cut into thin slices. Stir until everything is melted, then add the pepper. Your fondue is ready. We recommend tasting it on country bread.

Why are we talking about a recipe, especially a high-calorie one? Well, first of all because it is, in our humble opinion, one of the best things on earth and we wanted to share it.

If you remember, when we introduced lipids, we already mentioned France which, despite having a typical cuisine particularly rich in saturated fats, has, on average, no high incidence of heart disease. The phenomenon is known as the French paradox and was first coined by a scholar of the University of Bordeaux, Serge Renaud[42]. Several hypotheses have been made about the explanation of the paradox; I leave it to you to find a solution after reading this chapter. I believe it will not be difficult for you, and I also believe that you will then enjoy your fondue even more.

We have seen how carbohydrates can be converted into fat by the body when needed. Let us not forget, however, that fats can also be taken, as they

---

[42] Ferrieres, J. (2004). "The French Paradox; Lessons for other countries". *Heart*. 90 (1): 107–111. PMC 1768013□. PMID 14676260. doi:10.1136/heart.90.1.107

are, from the diet. Let's see how our body treats the lipids contained in that delicious cheese we have just devoured.

The digestion of lipids takes place mainly at the exit of the stomach. Here, fats are attacked by bile, produced by the liver, which emulsifies them, i.e. it breaks them down into many small droplets, to allow enzymes to attack them better. And enzymes are not long in coming: lipase, produced by the pancreas and the walls of the intestine, breaks down lipids into their components, which, if you remember, are glycerol and fatty acids. These substances, through the walls of the intestine, do not enter the bloodstream as carbohydrates do, but rather the lymphatic system. This circulatory system is a "twin" system of the bloodstream, much lesser-known, that runs through the whole of our body, with the task of draining excess water from the tissues and sending it back into the bloodstream, transporting our white blood cells and, indeed, transporting some molecules introduced with food.

Fatty acids, however, cannot travel within body fluids as they are. The reason is the same for which if you pour a tablespoon of oil into a glass of water it remains separate: the fats are insoluble in liquids. For this reason, you need certain proteins (called lipoproteins) which work a bit like buses. In order to board these means of transport, due to their structure, fatty acids and glycerol must be temporarily re-assembled, forming an old acquaintance of ours: triglycerides. The lipoproteins that take the lipids from the "bus stop" of the small intestine are called chylomicrons[43].

On board their bus-lipoprotein chylomicron, triglycerides happily travel into the vessels of the lymphatic system. After a full-fat meal, our lymph is well dense and whitish for all these lipids, like liquid cream. The lymph then flows into the bloodstream, and from there the bus-lipoproteins carry their fat content to those who need it, that is to say to the cells of the muscles (to produce energy, with the process we have already seen) and to the fat cells (to store them). Once at their destination, the triglycerides are again broken down into fatty acids and glycerol (in our visualization, they "get off" the bus), and enter the cells.

---

[43] David L. Nelson and Michael M. Cox, Lehninger Principles of Biochemistry 6th Edition

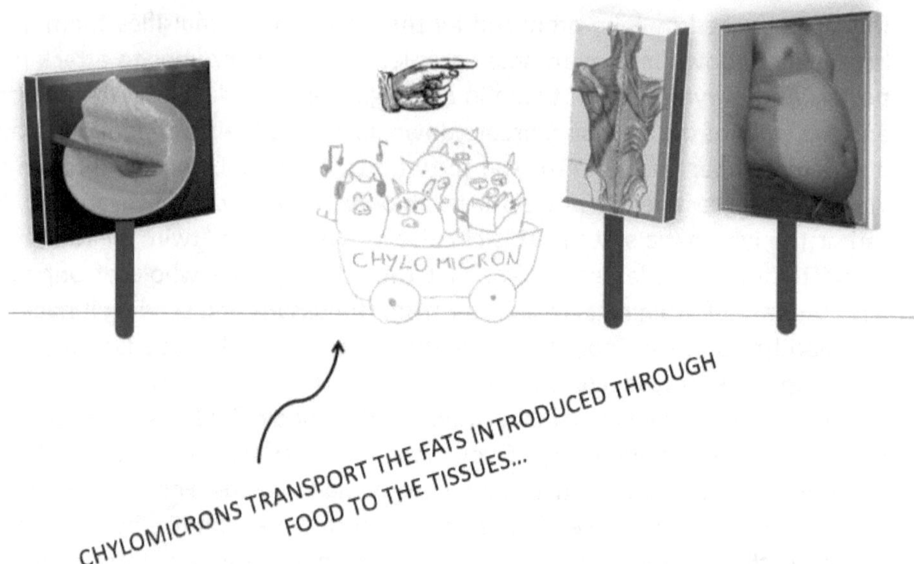

We also saw, while talking about carbohydrates, that triglycerides can appear in the body without being introduced with food, remember? This happens when the liver produces them from scratch starting with acetyl-coenzyme A. In this case, as well, lipids need a "bus"-lipoprotein to travel. This time, the name is different: the means of transport that starts from the liver is called VLDL (Very Low-Density Lipoprotein)[44]. The destination, as we know, is our beloved fatty tissue flab.

Cholesterol and the Allied Planes

If there was a survey on the less popular organic molecules, cholesterol would beat everyone. Accused over the years of all sorts of atrocity, it is

---

[44] Gibbons GF, Wiggins D, Brown AM, Hebbachi AM (2004). "Synthesis and function of hepatic very-low-density lipoprotein.". *Biochem Soc Trans*. 32 (Pt 1): 59–64. PMID 14748713. doi:10.1042/bst0320059

considered some kind of poison contained in bacon which pollutes our blood tests, leading us to sure death. It is therefore worthwhile to provide some clarity: perhaps, once again, there is someone being wrongly accused.

Cholesterol is considered a lipid because it is insoluble in water, and in organic chemistry this is the property which identifies fats. Its molecular structure, however, is different from that of the triglycerides we have encountered, of which it is merely a distant relative[45].

Most of the cholesterol in our body (70 to 90 percent!) is not taken with food but produced by the enzymes of all the cells in our body. The starting point is an old friend of ours: acetyl-coenzyme A. Starting from three of these molecules, through a long series of successive chemical reactions, comes a molecule of cholesterol.

But why does our body bother to produce this nefarious substance? The reason is that it is all but harmful: actually, it is essential to our lives. Cholesterol is in fact, first, a fundamental component of the cell membrane. All the cells have it, and besides protecting them it is used to decide who to let in or out and how. Without it, the cell would be like a house without walls. So, without cholesterol, there would simply be no life.

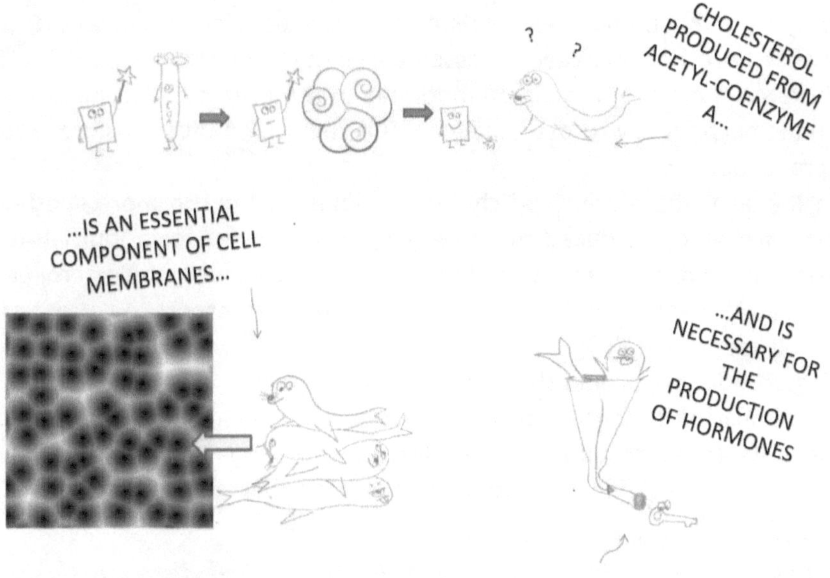

---

[45] Cholesterol at the US National Library of Medicine Medical Subject Headings (MeSH)

Moreover, cholesterol is the basis for the production of many hormones (which, as we have seen, are indispensable for the regulation of the body's reactions) and is indispensable for the production of bile[46]. There is no "good cholesterol" or "bad cholesterol": cholesterol is not Mr. Jekyll and Dr. Hide; it is one and only one. The misunderstanding stems from the excessive simplification of the path that cholesterol makes in our body. So, let's try to shed some light on this.

We have seen that all lipids, being insoluble in liquids, need a means to travel in the blood and other fluids of our body: the "buses"-lipoproteins. Cholesterol is no exception: he also needs to bind himself to lipoproteins to travel. The cholesterol we eat (red meat, eggs and dairy products are rich in cholesterol), once in the intestine, gets in line with the triglyceride relatives, and climbs on the "buses"-lipoprotein called chylomicrons. However, it is not allowed to go down, together with the triglycerides, to the "stops" of adipose tissue and muscles: cholesterol must remain, calm and silent, until the "end of the route", that is, the liver.

Indeed, the liver is the center of the management of cholesterol in the body. We have seen, in fact, that all our cells produce it, but it is the liver that produces the most, and then sends it into the blood for the benefit of those cells that have not managed to assemble enough for their needs. The food cholesterol, therefore, remains temporarily in the liver, so that the latter can see how much "ready to use" cholesterol is there, and thus possibly reducing the production.

In the liver, therefore, food cholesterol joins that (much more substantial, as we have seen) produced by the organ, and prepares for a journey to the cells that need it, throughout the body. In this case as well, cholesterol gets in line with triglycerides, and uses the same means of transport to get out of the liver: the lipoprotein VLDL.

Triglycerides are always the first to "get off"; when the bus-lipoprotein VLDL has lost most of its triglycerides and therefore mainly contains cholesterol, it changes its structure and becomes LDL (low density lipoprotein). LDL now focuses on transporting cholesterol to the cells that need it[47]. For instance,

---

[46] *Sadava D, Hillis DM, Heller HC, Berenbaum MR (2011). Life: The Science of Biology 9th Edition. San Francisco: Freeman. pp. 105–114. ISBN 1-4292-4646-4.*

[47] Dashti M, Kulik W, Hoek F, Veerman EC, Peppelenbosch MP, Rezaee F (2011). "A phospholipidomic analysis of all defined human plasma lipoproteins.". *Sci*

testicles may need cholesterol to produce male sex hormones. Or, the damaged wall of a blood vessel may need it, cholesterol being one of the main constituents of cell membranes.

But the epic of cholesterol transport does not end here: there is another class of lipoproteins, called HDL (high density lipoprotein)[48]. Its role is to collect the excess cholesterol that is wandering through the blood vessels: in fact, this lipid is not always used completely, and frequently there is excess. The HDL-bus picks up these cholesterol molecules and returns them to the liver, which either recycles them or uses them to produce bile (which is also the method for removing cholesterol from the body: bile, in fact, joins the residues of digested food to form the feces).

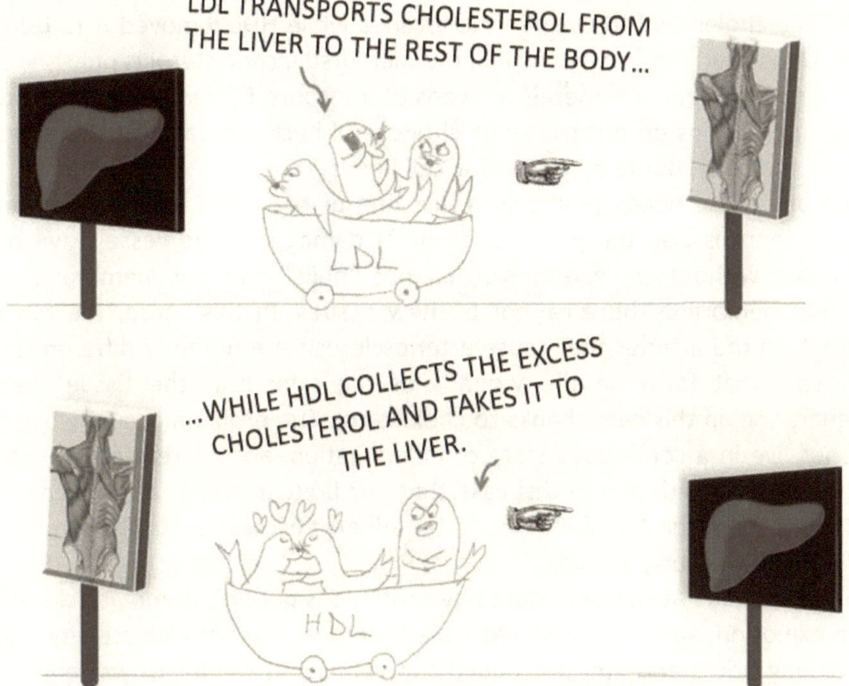

Let's think about it for a moment: if cholesterol was a toxic substance, would our body worry about bringing it back to the liver for reuse via HDLs?

Rep. 1 (139). PMC 3216620□. PMID 22355656. doi:10.1038/srep00139

[48] *Betteridge; et al. (2008). "Structural requirements for PCSK9-mediated degradation of the low-density lipoprotein receptor". PNAS. 105 (35): 13045–13050. doi:10.1073/pnas.0806312105.*

The reason why high cholesterol levels are typically associated with an increased risk of cardiovascular disease is that excess cholesterol, if not collected by HDLs, can tend to settle on the walls of the arteries, causing them to lose elasticity and forming a plaque that tends to swell; more or less the same as when dirt clogs the sink tube: water flows slowly and with difficulty.

In the case of arteriosclerosis, it is the blood that circulates with the most fatigue in the body, causing suffering in vital organs such as the brain, heart and kidneys. If neglected, arteriosclerosis can lead to total vessel occlusion or blood loss. These are terrible situations that evoke death solely by their name: heart attack, stroke, angina, thrombosis...

For years, HDL has been called "the good cholesterol" and LDL "the bad cholesterol"; this is because, due to an excessive simplification, LDL was said to cause the cholesterol to occlude the arteries while HDL removed it to bring it back to the liver... In fact, we now know that, firstly, cholesterol is only one and the two lipoproteins are merely a means of transport. Moreover, we know that these lipoproteins do not transport cholesterol back and forth just to show it around the body, but to meet specific cell needs.

Among these needs (and this is just one of the examples we mentioned earlier) there is also the periodic repair of damaged blood vessels: we have seen that without cholesterol you cannot "build" the cell membrane, and without membrane there cannot be new tissues. In this sense, the famous plaques on the arteries that cause arteriosclerosis are not very different from the scars that form on the wounds of the skin: it is the tissue that is regenerating, in this case thanks to cholesterol. The problem occurs when the arteries live in a continuous state of inflammation, and therefore need to be constantly repaired. It is in this case that our body is urged to produce more and more cholesterol, and that the latter adheres excessively to the arteries by widening the existing plaques.

Imagine a city at war devastated by continuous periodic bomb attacks. After each explosion, some allied planes parachute over the unfortunate city crates containing bricks and lime to rebuild the damage in the destroyed buildings. The problem is that some of these crates end up where they shouldn't, blocking the water channels that are essential for city life. The warring city is your body with constant inflammation, the brick crates are the cholesterol needed to rebuild it, and the water channels are the blocked arteries.

For years, the solution has been thought to be a reduction in cholesterol (by eating less foods containing cholesterol, or by taking drugs that inhibit cholesterol production). This is tantamount, in our warring city, to shooting down allied planes carrying crates of bricks. In the very short term, this may seem like a sensible solution: no more crates fall into the precious channels. However, some problems are beginning to arise in the medium term.

First, it happens that the allied command sees, via satellite, that the city is not being reconstructed. Knowing nothing but this, it gives the order to intensify the sending of bricks. As a result, many more planes arrive than we can shoot down, and we are back to square one. This scenario corresponds to the attempt to introduce less cholesterol with food. If you remember, most cholesterol does not come from outside, but is produced by our own body from the dear, old acetyl-coenzyme A. If our body thinks that it needs more cholesterol, the fact that we reduce that small percentage taken with food does not really bother it. Simply, it increases its autonomous production. Well, yes: eating less food containing cholesterol does not lower it[49]. Let's say, however, that our anti-aircraft artillery is effective enough to shoot down a huge number of friendly planes. This is the case if we take drugs that, in fact, chemically reduce the cholesterol produced.

It does not take a great deal of imagination to figure out where the problem lies: shooting down the planes of the allies prevents us from properly rebuilding our city. Let us remember that cholesterol is necessary for life: if it is too low, the body does not function properly. Some studies, for instance, have shown a clear correlation between low levels of cholesterol achieved artificially and diseases such as cancer[50], Parkinson's disease[51], depression[52] and very serious personality changes[53].

---

[49] Handbook of Nutrition and Food, Second Edition, a cura di Carolyn D. Berdanier,Johanna T. Dwyer,Elaine B. Feldman

[50] Clinical Research: Statins And Toxicity | July 2007, "Effect of the Magnitude of Lipid Lowering on Risk of Elevated Liver Enzymes, Rhabdomyolysis, and Cancer" Insights From Large Randomized Statin Trials, Alawi A. Alsheikh-Ali, MD; Prasad V. Maddukuri, MD; Hui Han, MD; Richard H. Karas, MD, PhD

[51] Mov Disord. 2008 May 15;23(7):1013-8. doi: 10.1002/mds.22013. Low LDL cholesterol and increased risk of Parkinson's disease: prospective results from Honolulu-Asia Aging Study, Huang X, Abbott RD, Petrovitch H, Mailman RB, Ross GW.

[52] Biol Psychol. Author manuscript; available in PMC 2011 May 1, published in final edited form as: , Biol Psychol. 2010 May; 84(2): 186–191.published online 2010 Jan 28. doi: 10.1016/j.biopsycho.2010.01.012 "Cholesterol, Triglycerides, and the Five-Factor Model of Personality", Angelina R. Sutin, Antonio Terracciano, Barbara Deiana, Manuela Uda, David Schlessinger, Edward G. Lakatta,and Paul T. Costa, Jr.

[53] Epidemiology. 2001 Mar;12(2):168-72.Low serum cholesterol concentration and risk of

So, what do we do? Perhaps we need a change of perspective: instead of raging about friendly planes, why don't we try to reduce or eliminate the terrorist attacks that underlie it all? Without attacks, the allied command has no reason to send so many planes, and without this continuous rain of crates our channels can function without problem. Translated into reality: by eliminating or reducing constant inflammation, the level of cholesterol automatically drops because there is no longer a continuous need for repairs. So, there is no growth of plaques, and it becomes possible for HDLs to progressively reduce existing ones[54].

The evidence is that research conducted by a Harvard team[55] has shown that measuring the amount of a particular protein, which is a mirror of the level of inflammation of the body, is much more effective than LDL as a "warning sign" for the risk of heart attacks and cardiovascular disease.

So, the right question to live healthy and long is not, "How can I lower my cholesterol?" But rather, "How can I reduce the level of inflammation in my body?" It is by eliminating terrorist attacks, and not allied planes, that the city can live and grow peacefully.

Inflammation, under normal conditions, is nothing more than our body's response to something irritating or harmful. However, various studies have shown that some substances introduced with food can, in the long run, cause an inflammatory state of the arteries, activating particular signal-molecules called cytokines, which in turn trigger the inflammatory process. Our body seems to react to these substances in the long run as if they were something toxic. In detail, according to very precise studies:

- the rapid increase in the concentration of blood sugar (caused, as we will see in detail below, to a great extent by sugars and refined cereals)[56] is a cause of inflammation.

---

suicide. Ellison LF, Morrison HI.

[54] The Great Cholesterol Myth: Why Lowering Your Cholesterol Won't Prevent Heart Disease-and the Statin-Free Plan That Will, Jonny Bowden, Stephen Sinatra, Fair Winds Press, 01 nov 2012

[55] Comparison of C-Reactive Protein and Low-Density Lipoprotein Cholesterol Levels in the Prediction of First Cardiovascular Events, Paul M. Ridker, M.D., Nader Rifai, Ph.D., Lynda Rose, M.S., Julie E. Buring, Sc.D., and Nancy R. Cook, Sc.D., N Engl J Med 2002; 347:1557-1565November 14, 2002DOI: 10.1056/NEJMoa021993

[56] Circulation. 2002 Oct 15;106(16):2067-72, Inflammatory cytokine concentrations are acutely increased by hyperglycemia in humans: role of oxidative stress, Esposito K, Nappo F, Marfella R, Giugliano G, Giugliano F, Ciotola M, Quagliaro L, Ceriello A, Giugliano D.

- the infamous trans fats[57] also have a strong inflammatory component.
- alcohol[58] and smoking[59], among their harmful effects, also cause persistent inflammation (not all commonplaces about cholesterol can be wrong, right?).

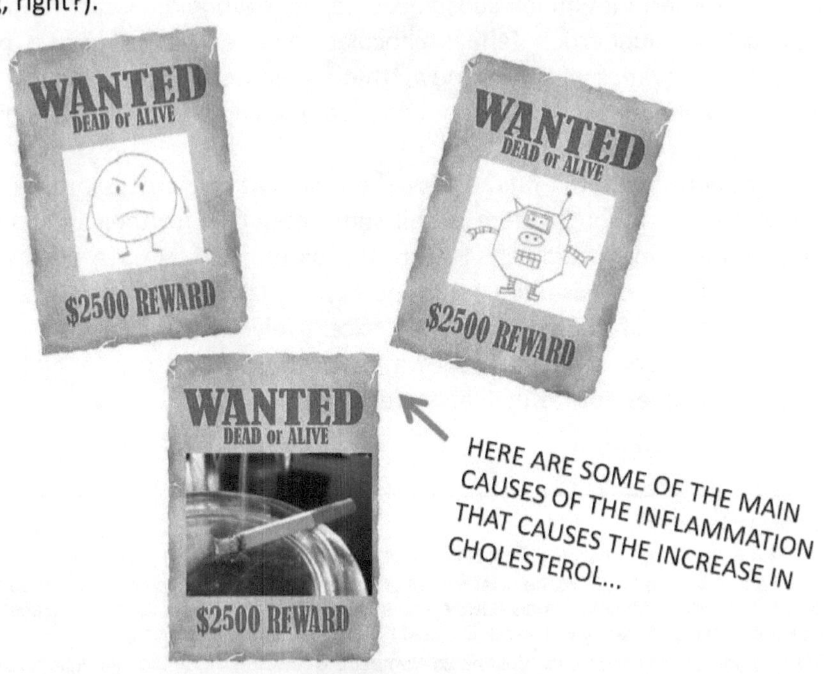

What instead can reduce the inflammatory state is:
- the consumption of fruit and vegetables: many studies[60] have shown[61] that the regular consumption of fresh fruit and vegetables at each meal leads to a reduction in the proteins that signal inflammation.

---

[57] Am J Clin Nutr. 2004 Apr;79(4):606-12, Dietary intake of trans fatty acids and systemic inflammation in women, Mozaffarian D, Pischon T, Hankinson SE, Rifai N, Joshipura K, Willett WC, Rimm EB.

[58] Alcohol and Inflammation & Immune Responses, Summary of the 2006 Alcohol and Immunology Research Interest Group (AIRIG) meeting, Thomas J. Waldschmidt, Robert T. Cook, and Elizabeth J. Kovacs

[59] Nohra Chalouhi, Muhammad S. Ali, Robert M. Starke, et al., "Cigarette Smoke and Inflammation: Role in Cerebral Aneurysm Formation and Rupture," Mediators of Inflammation, vol. 2012, Article ID 271582, 12 pages, 2012. doi:10.1155/2012/271582

[60] The American Journal of Clinical Nutrition, November 2005 , vol. 82 no. 5 1052-1058, A 4-wk intervention with high intake of carotenoid-rich vegetables and fruit reduces plasma C-reactive protein in healthy, nonsmoking men, Bernhard Watzl, Sabine E Kulling, Jutta Möseneder, Stephan

- a diet rich in polyunsaturated fats of the type Omega 3[62], which we have already discussed (while Omega 6 probably slows down their beneficial action).

- the consumption of substances called flavonoids, which abound in foods such as blueberries, fennel, chocolate and red wine. The last two, of course, in moderation: it is well known that a glass of good red wine every now and then is good for the heart, and with regard to chocolate, we speak of a few squares of dark chocolate[63].

What about saturated fats? As for the inflammatory process, research has cleared them[64], although there is still some doubt about their inflammatory effects in overweight people[65]. Historically, saturated fats have been blamed for causing heart disease due to an increase in LDL lipoproteins when foods rich in this type of fat are introduced excessively. In fact, not only one, but many studies over time have shown that, in the long run, a diet rich in saturated fats does not result in an increase in LDL[66] [67] [68] [69].

W Barth, Achim Bub

[61] The American Journal of Clinical Nutrition June 2006_ vol. 83_no. 6_1369-1379, "Dietary patterns are associated with biochemical markers of inflammation and endothelial activation in the Multi-Ethnic Study of Atherosclerosis (MESA)" , Jennifer A Nettleton, Lyn M Steffen, Elizabeth J Mayer-Davis, Nancy S Jenny,Rui Jiang, David M Herrington, David R Jacobs Jr

[62] Nutrition in Clinical Practice Volume 25 Number 6 December 2010, Diet and Inflammation Leo Galland, MD

[63] Nutrition in Clinical Practice Volume 25 Number 6 December 2010, Diet and Inflammation Leo Galland, MD

[64] "Relationships between serum fatty acid composition and multiple markers of inflammation and endothelial function in an elderly population", Petersson, Helena et al., Atherosclerosis , Volume 203 , Issue 1 , 298 - 303

[65] Diabetes Care. 2003 May;26(5):1362-8, "Insulin resistance, inflammation, and serum fatty acid composition", Fernández-Real JM, Broch M, Vendrell J, Ricart W.

[66] Br Med J. 1963 Mar 2; 1(5330): 571–576; "Diet and Plasma Cholesterol in 99 Bank Men"; J. N. Morris, Jean W. Marr, J. A. Heady, G. L. Mills, and T. R. E. Pilkington

[67] Am J Clin Nutr. 1976 Dec;29(12):1384-92; "Daily nutritional intake and serum lipid levels. The Tecumseh study", Nichols AB, Ravenscroft C, Lamphiear DE, Ostrander LD Jr.

[68] Am J Clin Nutr. 1965 Feb;16:238-42; "THE RELATIONSHIP OF NUTRIENT INTAKE AND EXERCISE TO SERUM CHOLESTEROL LEVELS IN WHITE MALES IN EVANS COUNTY, GEORGIA" STULB SC, MCDONOUGH JR, GREENBERG BG, HAMES CG.

[69] Israel Journal of Medical Science,. 1969 Nov-Dec;5(6):1117-27; "Serum cholesterol: its distribution and association with dietary and other variables in a survey of 10,000 men", Kahn HA, Medalie JH, Neufeld HN, Riss E, Balogh M, Groen JJ.

This does not surprise us: if a substance does not cause inflammation, in the long run it does not cause a hyper-production of cholesterol.

Remember Dr. Keys who abhorred saturated fatty acids? We have just seen and explained in detail why it is not true. This does not mean, of course, that we can feed on eggs and lard (we will see later the ideal proportions between the various nutrients in a diet), but it certainly shows that there has been an over-demonization of these foods.

The real enemies of your heart and cardiovascular system, we now know, are trans oils, sugars and refined cereals. And their best friends are fresh fruits and vegetables, dried fruit, whole grains, and sometimes a good glass of red wine and a square of dark chocolate, all rich in the substances we listed above[70].

---

[70] J Am Coll Cardiol. 2006 Aug 15;48(4):677-85. Epub 2006 Jul 24; "The effects of diet on inflammation: emphasis on the metabolic syndrome"; Giugliano D, Ceriello A, Esposito K

9. The Metabolism of Proteins

"A protein molecule is like a string of beads, each bead being an amino acid"
Neal Barnard

The Body That Eats Itself

We already know that proteins have a fundamental role as "bricks" and "gears" of our whole body. Unfortunately, proteins tend to get damaged quite easily, and must be replaced continuously for tissues and organs to continue to exist and function; this normal process is called protein turnover[71].

The average life span of proteins depends on the type: it ranges from less than two hours for enzymes and hormones, to several days for proteins with more structural function. It is a huge job for our body: it would be as if the bricks of a house had to be replaced one by one every week, or if the gears of a clock had to be changed ten times a day!

A small protein, called ubiquitin, has the function of "inspector": it identifies the degraded proteins, which are no longer able to carry out their function, and "labels" them, binding to them. Subsequently, various specific enzymes dismantle the labelled proteins, releasing the individual amino acids that formed them.

Problems in the functioning of ubiquitin are associated with many diseases (neurodegenerative diseases, cystic fibrosis, cancers...); imagine a car that does not undergo any servicing for years and years, and you will easily understand why.

Our body, which never throws anything away, recycles the amino acids released in this way and which are still usable for the formation of new proteins. The amino acids that derive from this recovery action, however, are not enough on their own: partly because a part of the original amino acids is lost with the degradation of proteins, partly because new ones are constantly required for the growth and development of cells and tissues. Therefore, it is essential to continuously introduce "fresh" proteins with the diet.

---

[71] *Thomas E Creighton (1993). Proteins: Structures and Molecular Properties (2nd ed.). W H Freeman and Company. ISBN 0-7167-2317-4.*

Protein digestion begins in the stomach, by means of an enzyme (pepsin) that starts to "break" the long chains of amino acids. Other enzymes in the small intestine then complete the process, and the individual amino acids are absorbed and enter the bloodstream, through which they reach the liver or tissues that need them[72].

It may happen that the diet introduces more amino acids than those needed, at present, for the turnover of proteins. Since it is not possible for our bodies to store amino acids, these must follow a different path.

First, some enzymes break each amino acid into two parts: one is called the amino group, and the other is called the carbon skeleton.

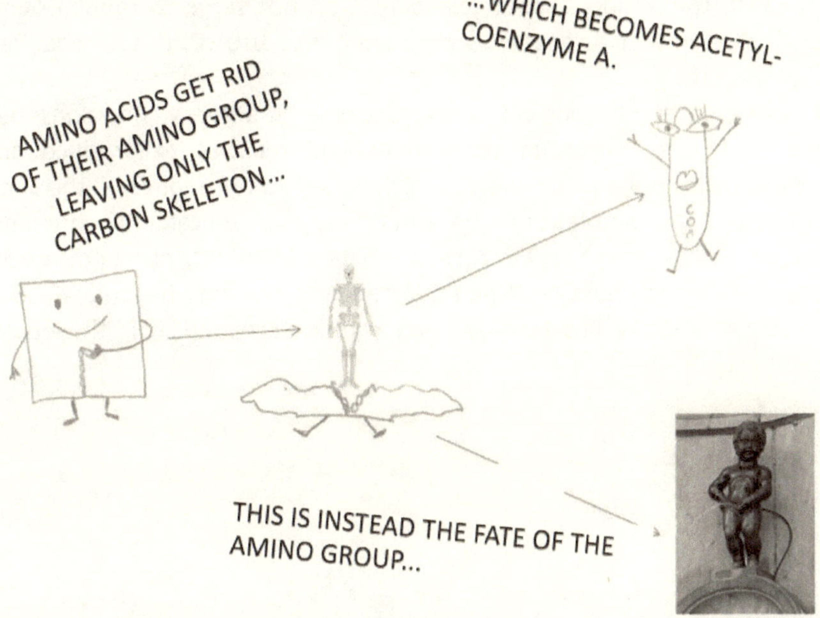

The amino group undergoes a series of very complex transformation processes. We are only interested in knowing (with some simplification) that the result of all these processes is a waste substance called urea, which is expelled from our body through urine.

The fate of carbon skeletons, on the other hand, depends on the type of initial amino acids; we can simplify this by saying that, among the main final

[72] Maton, Anthea; Jean Hopkins; Charles William McLaughlin; Susan Johnson; Maryanna Quon Warner; David LaHart; Jill D. Wright (1993). Human Biology and Health. Englewood Cliffs, New Jersey, USA: Prentice Hall. ISBN 0-13-981176-1. OCLC 32308337.

products, we find two of our acquaintances: pyruvate and acetyl CoA. We already know that these substances are combustible for our mitochondria, or the basis to produce fats. It is therefore clear how energy can be derived from amino acids, as well as from carbohydrates and fats[73].

This reaction can, in some cases, also work in reverse: our body can synthesize amino acids, when these are not introduced through food, starting with substances such as pyruvate. Be careful though: this is not possible for all amino acids. If you remember, there are certain types of amino acids, called essential, which must necessarily be introduced with food. They are precisely those that cannot be synthesized by the body.

In short: the amino acids ingested that do not serve to rebuild our body through the protein turnover become energy to use or, if not used, reserve energy (i.e. fat...)

One last note: our body can, under extreme emergency conditions, use the amino acids that make up the tissues and muscles to produce energy. However, this is done when there is nothing left to burn: once all the supplies, including glycogen and fat ones, have been used up, we can only obtain energy from the body's own tissues. After running out of fat, our body begins to metabolize its own muscles. When this happens, the limit beyond which a diet is no longer healthy has already been widely exceeded. It is the body that "eats" itself.

---

[73] Michael Lieberman, Allan D. Marks, *Biochimica medica*, Casa Editrice Ambrosiana, 2014, ISBN 978-88-08-18217-3

10.   Insulin and Glucagon

The Tragic End of the Greedy Senator

In his novel, *Buddenbrooks: The Decline of a Family*, Thomas Mann tells of an old diabetic man whose passion for sweets goes a bit too far:

"James Mollendorpf, the oldest of the merchant senators, died in a grotesque and horrible way. The instinct of self-preservation became very weak in this diabetic old man, and in the last years of his life he fell a victim to a passion for cakes and pastries. Dr. Grabow, as Mollendorpf's family physician, had protested energetically, and the distressed relatives employed gentle constraint to keep the head of the family from committing suicide with sweet bake-stuffs. But the old Senator, mental wreck as he was, rented a room somewhere, in some convenient street, like Little Groping Alley, or Angelswick, or Behind-The Wall, a little hole of a room, whither he would secretly betake himself to consume sweets. And there they found his lifeless body, the mouth still full of half-masticated cake, the crumbs upon his coat and upon the wretched table. A mortal stroke had supervened, and put a stop to slow dissolution".

The miserable end of Mr. James, besides serving as a sure warning against the instinct to grab a second serving of dessert, reminds us (perhaps in a somewhat grotesque way) how much sugar plays a crucial role in the quality of our lives. To fully understand this theme, however, we need to delve into the connections of metabolism with some hormones of our body. Without these pieces of the puzzle (also connected to diabetes, the terrible disease from which poor Mr. James suffered), it is not possible to really understand the effect that some foods have on our body.

Let's start with a definition: the concentration of simple sugars in a person's blood is called glycemia: the higher the glycemia, the more glucose (or other simple sugars) are present in our blood. In healthy people, glycemia on an empty stomach is usually between 60 and 99 milligrams of sugar per deciliter of blood. This value rises to 130-150 after meals, when the sugars absorbed by the intestine enter the bloodstream[74].

In general, our body is quite "anxious" about glycemia, and has activated numerous mechanisms to control and regulate it. The reason is that it represents a serious danger both when it is too high and when it is too low. Too little blood sugar and too much blood sugar are both lethal to the body.

The reason why having little sugar in circulation (hypoglycemia) is dangerous is easily said: The brain has a continuous need to "burn" sugars to function, so much so that almost 60% of the glucose in circulation in the blood is used by our nervous system.

Since the brain is not able to store glucose in any way, there must always be a minimum amount in the blood. Otherwise it will slow down and then go out like a car on empty: this means symptoms ranging from headaches, fatigue and drowsiness to convulsions, fainting and coma.

Reading this, one could say that it is preferable for the body to have a lot, a very lot of sugar circulating in the blood. Unfortunately, however, even the opposite condition (hyperglycemia, i.e. too many sugars in the bloodstream) is very dangerous. Why?

In excessive quantities, glucose is a toxic substance: It damages the inner wall of blood vessels, forming plaques that prevent blood circulation (arteriosclerosis). This also causes very serious damage to certain organs such as the kidneys, brain, heart and eyes; it can also cause ulcers and wounds to the skin that do not heal[75].

The issue of the right amount of blood sugar (not too much, not too little) therefore seems quite delicate. For this reason, we have two sentinel-hormones: glucagon and insulin, both produced by the pancreas.

These two sentinels have opposite functions:

•	glucagon corrects situations where glycemia is too low, which means scarcity of blood sugars.

•	insulin, on the other hand, handles situations where levels of glycemia are too high, i.e. excess blood sugars.

---

[74] ADA Standards of Medical Care in Diabetes, 2016

[75] Glucose Toxicity, George Fantus, M.D.Senior Scientist, Division of Cellular & Molecular Biology, Toronto General Research Institute (TGRI), Mount Sinai Hospital, Toronto, ON, CANADA, ac.no.irhsm@sutnaf, Last Update: May 20, 2009.

Let's start by observing the insulin in action. It's Sunday, you've just had a binge, and now you're resting on the couch with your belly full. But inside you it's far from quiet... as soon as the carbohydrates from that delicious cheesecake enter the bloodstream in the form of simple sugars, your glycemia rises.

The pancreas (a large gland under the stomach) has inside some cells, called Beta cells, which are activated when glycemia rises, and react by releasing insulin into the bloodstream.

We already know that each hormone is a "key" that activates a certain "lock". Let's see which locks trigger the insulin.

First, the hormone activates receptors that are found on the cell membranes of muscles (including the heart) and adipose tissues. What happens when the lock "clicks"?

If you remember, we had already met the Gluts, the "tourist-catchers" of glucose. The Glut takes glucose from the blood and introduces it into the cell by making it cross the membrane. Not all Gluts, however, are the same.

In particular, those working on the membranes of tissue cells, such as the nervous system, the retina or the testicles, work tirelessly with no need to be activated by nearly anything: It is enough for a molecule of glucose to pass next to it, in the bloodstream, to grab it and introduce it into the cell, towards its burning destiny. This is because these tissues are particularly dependent on glucose, since there is nothing else that they can use to produce energy (they cannot therefore "burn" fatty acids).

The Gluts of muscle cells and adipose tissue, instead, need the key-insulin to activate. Without it, they remain dormant[76].

Thanks to this mechanism, when there is little glucose in the blood you are sure that it will be used by the brain and other tissues that have no other choice. This prevents us, for instance, from fainting or going into a coma during the night, when blood glucose is limited as we do not eat for several hours. Only when glycemia rises, resulting in insulin production, do the muscle Gluts activate, and consequently they can participate in the banquet, after the neediest tissues have served themselves.

---

[76] Arthur C. Guyton, John E. Hall. Fisiologia medica. Elsevier srl, 2006. p. 966 ISBN 8821429369]

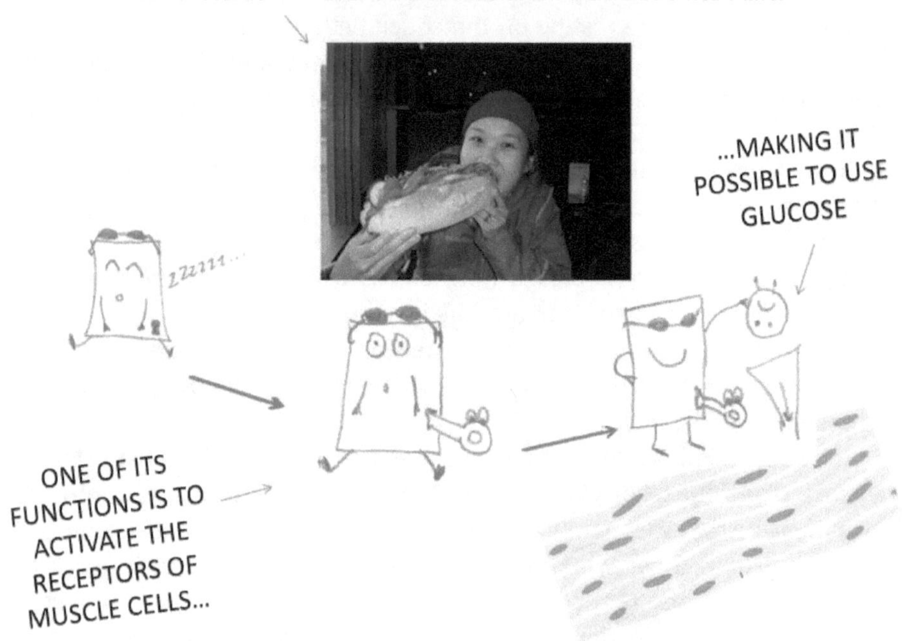

A note about the liver: this organ has another type of Glut, which is independent from insulin but gets activated by the simple presence of glucose, beyond a certain level, in the blood. In this way, the liver can independently carry out its work as a "storekeeper" of glucose (transforming it into glycogen, as you certainly remember). Moreover, the liver Gluts are the only ones to act as "bouncers" as well as "tourist-catchers": they can, indeed, put glucose back into the bloodstream, just like they introduced it into the cell. The glucose that enters the other tissues, in fact, no longer comes out. The liver, instead, is a generous warehouse: it accumulates glycogen for everyone and releases it for everyone. The glycogen stored by a muscle cell is solely for it.

Let's get back to insulin, though. A second mechanism activated by this hormone is the formation of glycogen. When it is inserted into the "locks" of liver and muscle cells, in fact, it activates a series of chemical reactions that allow the enzyme glycogen-synthesis to patiently sew the molecules of glucose to each other, forming the chains of glycogen. Insulin, therefore, does not limit itself to favoring the entry of glucose into these two types of cells, but also helps them to store it.

The third action of insulin concerns fats. In the liver and adipose tissue, it stimulates enzymes that produce fatty acids (the basis for triglycerides) from the acetyl-enzyme CoA and inhibits the enzyme lipase, which "disassembles" the triglycerides into fatty acids and glycerol, preparing their demobilization. In short, insulin makes it easier to produce fat and harder to dispose of it.

The three main tasks of insulin make perfect sense, if you consider the mandate given to it by the body, which is to dispose of excess glucose in the blood. Insulin fulfils this task in every possible way: by facilitating its entry into the cells, by favoring its accumulation (in the form of glycogen and fatty acids) and by hindering the use of fats as an energy source (by blocking lipase), so that glucose is burned.

Diabetics find themselves in a situation where insulin does not perform its function, either because the body does not produce enough of it, or because the "locks" it should trigger do not work properly. The consequence is hyperglycemia, i.e. the presence of too much glucose in the blood, with all the excess sugar damage we have seen (deficit in the nervous system, kidney problems, eye and cardiovascular problems). In addition, diabetics have problems getting sugar in to produce energy (remember the Gluts?), and this explains the lack of energy and exhaustion caused by the disease. Insulin injections allow diabetics to live a normal life, restoring the balance of blood sugar[77].

Finally, it should be noted that the rapid drop in blood sugar resulting from the work of insulin "ignites" some receptors of our nervous system which become alarmed and, for this reason, stimulate our hunger. That's why after a sweet snack you risk having a very sudden grumbling in the stomach.

Now, let's see what glucagon does. It's spring, and you are taking advantage of the sun to do a nice outdoor run. It may be the music at full volume, it may be the pleasure of running in the green, but today you are really outdoing yourself, so much so that you hardly notice how much your stomach grumbles, since at breakfast you had something very light. What is happening in your body?

---

[77] Diabetes Fact sheet N°312". *WHO*. October 2013. Archived from the original on 26 August 2013. Retrieved 25 March 2014.

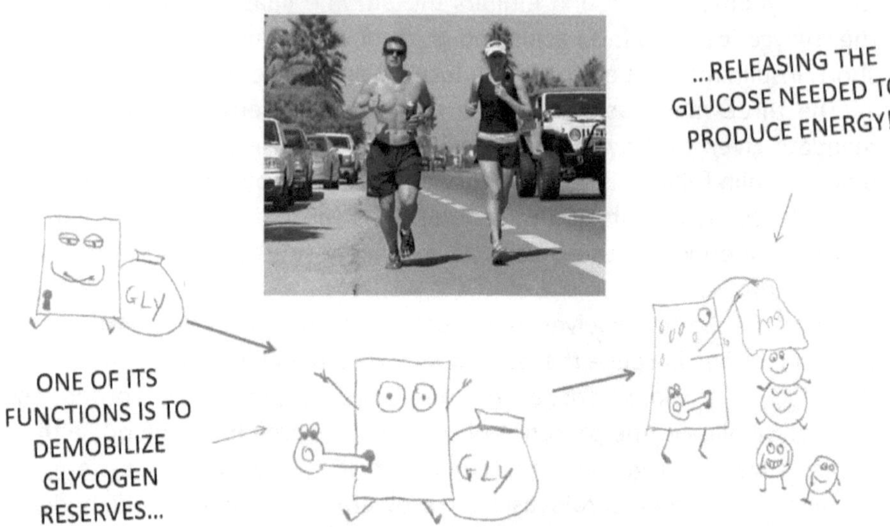

The little sugar in the bloodstream has already been consumed, the pancreas realizes that glycemia is low through its Alpha cells and produces glucagon. The mandate that the body gives to this hormone is simple: demobilize the stocks, make available as soon as possible something that the hungry mitochondria of the cells can burn. In order to fulfil its task, glucagon binds to its receptors in liver cells, and here stimulates the division of glycogen into glucose molecules and their release into the bloodstream. In addition, in adipose tissue, glucagon stimulates the transformation of triglycerides into glycerol and fatty acids, which are released into the blood (on board a new carrier: the protein albumin), available to produce energy.

It is therefore clear how, by "pulling the strings" of the two hormones insulin and glucagon, our body organizes the various metabolic activities according to the needs of the moment. However, this mechanism may jam...

Obese in Paradise

In the heart of the South Pacific Ocean lies the Tonga archipelago, a true earthly paradise of crystal-clear water, white beaches and lush nature with a wonderful perennial summer.

The inhabitants of this wonderful corner of the world, however, have a sad record: with 92% of the population over 30 overweight, Tonga is the fattest nation in the world. About 20% of the indigenous people suffer from diabetes, and death from issues related to over-feeding is ten times greater than in the UK.

This unfortunate condition, which affects many other islands in the Pacific, is largely caused by the change in diet that the advent of Western modernity has brought here: the traditional diet, rich in meat, fish, fresh fruits and vegetables, has slowly been replaced by a diet rich in packaged foods imported from outside, in parallel with the abandonment of agriculture. Over time, the purchase of food from abroad has become, in these countries isolated for centuries, a sign of social distinction. It is said that the wives of the first missionaries convinced the local women that the healthiest way to prepare meals for their families was to cook cakes in the Western way, in a real form of food colonialism. Now, the local diet is largely composed of canned foods, refined sugars and flours, sugary drinks and beer; the physical distance of the islands from other nations tends to favor long-life industrial foods to the disadvantage of fresh ones[78].

What happens in a body attacked by those junk foods that have transformed the population of Tonga, goes beyond the mechanisms we described above. The excess of insulin caused by the continuous presence of sugars in the blood, in fact, triggers a "sick" mechanism to which our body is very little prepared to respond. Let's not forget that, from an evolutionary point of view, very little time has passed since we were cave dwellers eating game. From this point of view, the level of preparation of our body to modern nutrition is not much different from that of the inhabitants of Tonga when, in the last century, they were tempted by the tarts of the missionaries.

Let's see what happens when glycemia is very often high in our blood. This condition is very common in modern societies; in fact, remember that all carbohydrates become simple sugars. If your diet is largely based on bread, crackers, bagels, rice, potatoes, pizza, biscuits, pasta, rice cakes.... You are most

---

[78] The Obesity Epidemic in the Pacific Islands, M i c h a e l C u r t i s, United States Department of Army, Journal of development and social transformation, Volume 1, November 2004

likely in this condition. Of course, sweets and all sugary foods also contribute to the glycemic emergency.

With this perennial abundance of blood sugar, the pancreas is extremely happy to continuously produce insulin in order to properly use and store the sweet glucose. With all this insulin in circulation, however, something happens to its cellular receptors, the "locks" that this hormone triggers.

Basically, our cells have a reaction mechanism to both deficiency and excess of certain substances. In general, when a substance that must produce certain reactions is scarce, the cell increases the number of receptors to be more likely to detect it. On the contrary, when the substance is too abundant, the cell reduces the number of receptors (let's imagine that it "plugs" some "locks") to hinder its effects.

If insulin is always in circulation, therefore, the cells tend to decrease the number of receptors on their membrane, becoming more resistant to the hormone (we talk about insulin-resistance). With fewer receptors, insulin is less effective in the performance of its tasks, and therefore glycemia in the blood struggles to drop. The pancreas keeps registering high glycemia and responds by producing even more insulin. As a result, cell receptors become even scarcer, in a loop that in the most serious cases leads to so-called type-two diabetes[79].

If you remember the effects of insulin on our body, it will also be clear what the devastating consequences of having this hormone continuously circulating can be: first, a greater quantity of fatty acids in circulation, with consequent ease of weight gain.

But not only: fat also accumulates in the liver, increasing the risk of liver steatosis (commonly called "fatty liver", and often a prelude to annoying inflammation or even cirrhosis), arteriosclerosis and other serious cardiovascular diseases (remember what causes plaques in the arteries?), hormonal imbalances and mood changes.

Moreover, paradoxically, insulin resistance leads to tiredness and loss of strength. This is because, due to the decrease in receptors on muscle cells, it is increasingly difficult to absorb glucose molecules. If you are always feeling tired, exhausted, lethargic and lacking in energy, ask yourself if there are not too many carbohydrates in your diet.

---

[79] Chiu HK, Tsai EC, Juneja R, et al. (August 2007). "Equivalent insulin resistance". *Diabetes Research and Clinical Practice*. 77: 237–44. PMID 17234296. doi:10.1016/j.diabres.2006.12.013

It is not surprising that some studies have revealed that a low presence of insulin in the blood is closely related to a high life expectancy[80]. Insulin, mind you, is not a poison per se. As we know, its fundamental task is substantially that of storing the excess nutrients as stock. Our ancestors who lived in caves would veer between periods of food abundance and periods of famine: had they not been able to store energy reserves within their bodies, our species would have become extinct very quickly. The problem arises when a mechanism toughened for the hard life of the Paleolithic finds itself managing our civilization of abundance of refined grains and sugars, as in the case of Tonga.

To stay young, fit and healthy, it is therefore essential to keep insulin under control. What can we do about this? Do we have to remove all carbohydrates from our lives? To answer this, we need to go into the concept of glycemic index.

The Truck and the Despotic Old Woman

In Woody Allen's comedy film, *Sleeper,* the body of a man who lived in the 1970s, and who had been cryogenically frozen by mistake after a duodenal ulcer operation, is found and defrosted in an America of the future. When the poor man wakes up, the doctors try to calm him down, and they do so in a peculiar way:

Doctor: "Here, smoke this. And be sure you get the smoke deep down into your lungs."

Woody Allen: "I don't smoke."

Doctor: "It's tobacco! It's one of the healthiest things for your body. Now, go ahead. You need all the strength you can get."

While it is quite unlikely that official medicine will in the future restore cigarettes, it is true that, with the passage of time, ideas on what is healthy and what is not have often changed, and it is precisely on this that the famous comedian was doing irony.

In the field of nutrition, we have already seen some of these changes, of course. For instance, the admission that there is no correlation between the

[80] Aging Dis. 2010 Oct; 1(2): 147–157., Published online 2010 Aug 26., PMCID: PMC3295030, Insulin, IGF-1 and longevity, Diana van Heemst[1,*]

cholesterol contained in the foods we eat and that in our blood, as we explained above. Also, in the past, there had been a collective love for margarine, the "good" antagonist of the "bad" butter, only to realize later that it was often full of the infamous hydrogenated fats.

There is another myth, however, that we want to address now. If you look through articles or statements from some time ago, it is not uncommon to find the assertion that complex carbohydrates, such as rice, pasta, bread (in short, cereals and their derivatives) provide "long-term energy" and are therefore always healthy for the diet, because they support us throughout the day. What is true about this assertion? There is a lot of confusion about this, and many conflicting opinions. Have we not just seen that an excess of carbohydrates causes deleterious changes to the normal cycle of insulin? Who is right?

For the sake of clarity, we need to start with a few definitions. Come on, they are essential for understanding. And, as always, we will try to give examples that can make them very easy.

Let's start with the glycemic index. It is a value that measures the speed with which the carbohydrates contained in a food flow into the bloodstream. Without going into the details of how it is calculated, it is enough to know that it is measured by a number, different for each food. The higher the number, the faster the carbohydrates contained in that food are absorbed after we eat it.

Up to 40, the glycemic index is considered very low; from 41 to 55, low; from 56 to 69, moderate and from 70 upwards, it is considered high. In Appendix D, you can find the glycemic indexes of the main foods[81].

In general, the presence in a food of different macronutrients, such as fiber, protein or fat, slows down the absorption of carbohydrates because it makes the work of the digestive system more difficult; this explains the low glycemic index of foods such as fruit, vegetables, milk or meat. The more, however, the carbohydrates are predominant or the only nutrients, the faster the absorption is and the glycemic index rises: see bread, pasta or cakes made with refined flour (while whole-meal flour, thanks to its fiber content, has a lower index).

Why should we be interested in this? It is immediate to link the concept of glycemic index to that of glycemia, and to think that the foods to be preferred are those with lower glycemic index: the "peaks" of sugar in the blood, in fact,

---

[81] Jenkins et al. *Glycemic index of foods: a physiological basis for carbohydrate exchange.* 1981, American Journal of Clinical Nutrition, Vol 34, 362-366

also cause peaks of insulin, with all the harmful effects that its massive presence in the blood causes. A distribution of the absorption of sugar more "spread" in the time, on the contrary, should avoid such peaks and, consequently, never cause an "over-insulinization" of the blood.

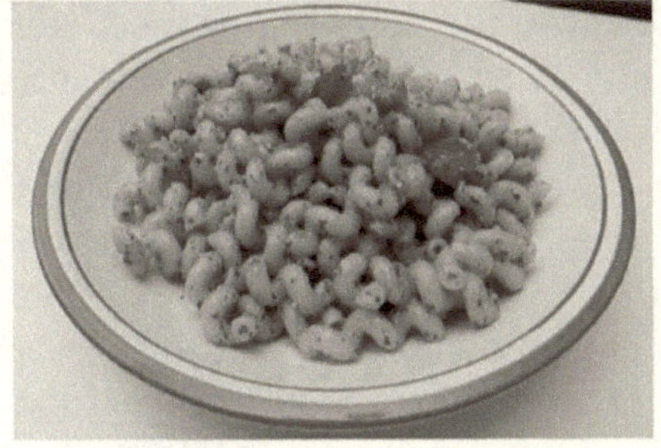

LARGE QUANTITIES OF FOODS WITH A HIGH GLYCEMIC INDEX CAUSE AN INCREASE IN THE AMOUNT OF INSULIN IN THE BLOOD.

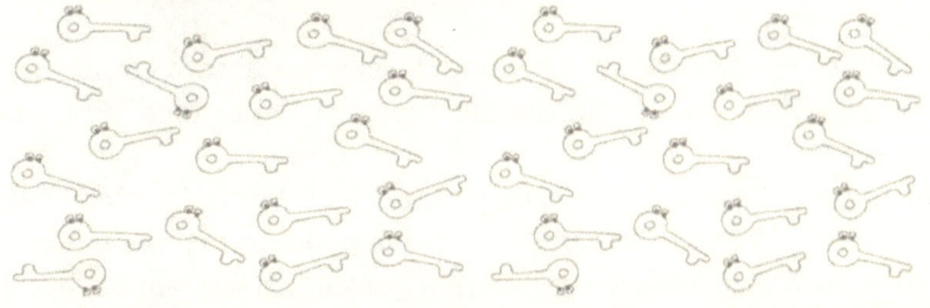

To make an analogy, let's imagine a truck with the tipper unloading its content, which represents our meal. Nearby lives an elderly woman who is very nervous and very sensitive to noise, and ready to shout and bark out of the window in proportion to the annoyance she feels. The vitriolic lady represents the beta cells of the pancreas, and the amount of screaming represents the amount of insulin they produce.

The glycemic index measures the speed at which the contents of the truck fall from the tipper and depends on what the truck is carrying. First, the vehicle unloads a content of gravel only, then one of gravel mixed with bitumen. The first load will fall quickly (high index); the second in a slower way, being more viscous (low index). The gravel represents the carbohydrates, and the bitumen the other macronutrients present in the food we are eating. A slice of white bread is like gravel: there is nothing to slow down the absorption of carbohydrates. An apricot is like gravel mixed with bitumen: the vegetable fibers that hold it together slow down the absorption of sugars.

The quicker the content drops, the more it makes noise, causing the screams of the sprightly granny. The first load will make a big noise, and will cause big screams: white bread will cause a rapid increase in glycemia, and therefore a consistent secretion of insulin.

In the case of the second load, however, the noise will be much less, and will only result in some mumbling. Just as an apricot only slightly increases glycemia, and thus causes marginal insulin secretion.

Is it really like that? Yes, but to a certain extent. Many diets or eating methods stop here. From a biochemical point of view, however, this is only the beginning.

Take for example the pumpkin (glycemic index 75) and milk chocolate (glycemic index 44). A comparison of the indexes would tell us that it is healthier to fill your belly with milk chocolate instead of pumpkin. Sadly, this is not the case.

It is necessary to consider not only how quickly we absorb carbohydrates, but also HOW MANY THERE ARE in the food, to understand how quickly glycemia rises.

Back to the old lady and the truck, it should be borne in mind that the annoyance and the resulting screams will also depend on the amount of load. We have seen how noisy the pure gravel that goes down fast can be, but if the load is only a few stones, the old lady won't be that much upset. On the other hand, even if the gravel mixed with bitumen is less noisy, if a hundred trucks arrive and continue to unload it throughout the afternoon, be sure that the lady will make herself heard loud and clear.

So: it's true that pumpkin carbohydrates are absorbed quickly and cause insulin peaks, but it's also true that there aren't many. The calculation of the glycemic load[82] therefore takes account of this: It multiplies the glycemic index of the pumpkin (75) by the grams of carbohydrates in one hundred grams of food (5.3 on average) divided by one hundred. The result is approximately 4.

If we do the same calculation for milk chocolate, we have: glycemic index (44) by the grams of carbohydrates in one hundred grams of food (on average about 80) divided by one hundred. The result is approximately 35. Much higher than the 4 of the pumpkin: in fact, even if the composition of the chocolate

---

[82] *European Journal of Clinical Nutrition* (2007) 61 (Suppl 1), S122–S131; doi:10.1038/sj.ejcn.1602942, Glycemic index and glycemic load: measurement issues and their effect on diet–disease relationships, B J Venn and T J Green

(which is rich in different ingredients) makes the carbohydrates more slowly assimilable than those of the pumpkin, it is also true that there are many more.

In the truck, there's a mixture that falls slower, but it's a lot, a lot more. Much more annoyance for the old lady, and much more screaming. A one hundred grams (3.5 ounces) of milk chocolate cause more insulin to be produced than a one hundred grams (3.5 ounces) of pumpkin; there vanishes the chocolate diet you had already envisioned.

Boiled carrots have a high glycemic index, close to that of glucose. But you can eat them with absolute peace of mind: even if carbohydrates are assimilated very quickly, they are too few to cause a significant peak in glycemia. There is pure gravel in the truck, but not enough to make noise.

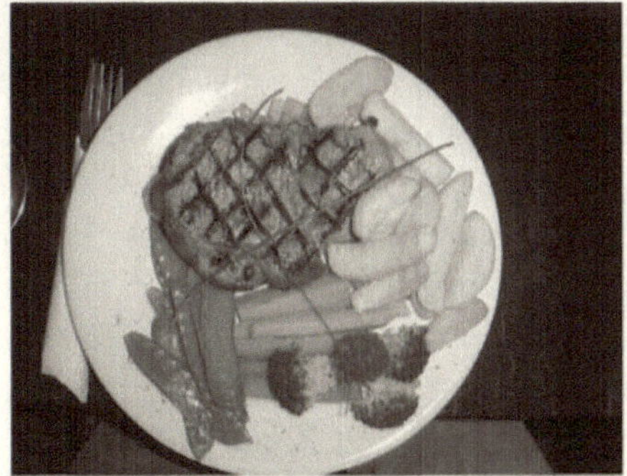

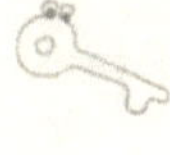

The glycemic load of a meal is considered low to 10, average between 10 and 20, and high over 20. If we want to keep the production of insulin under control, with all the benefits that this brings for health, longevity and weight control, we must therefore try to keep the glycemic load of each meal below 10, below the threshold that makes the old sprightly lady excessively nervous.

For each food, it is possible to calculate the quantity that can be eaten at once without the glycemic load exceeding the value of ten. In our metaphor, for each type of load (mixture of more or less gravel and more or less bitumen), it is possible to calculate the maximum allowed truck content, beyond which the old lady begins to rant and rave.

For those who want to try their hand at mathematics, the details of reasoning are at the end of Appendix D. It is enough, however, to know the rule that is derived from it: by dividing the glycemic load of a food by one thousand, you get the maximum amount that you can eat in a meal without the glycemic load exceeding ten. This allows insulin to be kept under control, with the enormous benefits that, as we know, derive from it in terms of weight control and general health[83].

For instance: coconut has a glycemic load of 3. One thousand divided by three makes 333, which means that eating up to about three hundred grams (12 ounces) of coconut, the glycemic load is under control.

If you make some calculations with the values in the table in Appendix D, you will see that there are foods for which the amount by which the threshold of ten is exceeded is really low. For instance, for white bread, it is about 18 grams (1000/56) and for biscuits about 15 grams (1000/63). Does this mean that we are forced to obsessively weigh these foods and eat their crumbs?

As always, you should let your commonsense guide you: it is not appropriate to become accountants of food and go to the restaurant armed with a calculator and table of glycemic loads. Insulin is not rat poison, and nothing happens in healthy people, if every now and then the glycemic load of a meal exceeds ten. The important thing is that it is not perpetually above this value. The table and the method of calculation should serve more as a guide and a warning, to understand which foods can be consumed without particular problems, to fill up, and which instead should be the subject of attention (you can eat them, but they cannot be the basis of the diet). I therefore invite you, out of curiosity, to try with some food: just to be aware of when your insulin production increases, and then handle this information without becoming obsessed with it.

In particular, here are some practical tips to help you control your glycemic load, and thus your insulin production:

• ensure that fruit and vegetables are never missing from your meals. These are foods that generally have a low glycemic load, so they can fill you up by making you consume less of them than foods with a high load. Wrap your

[83] Carbohydrate Counting, Glycemic Index, and Glycemic Load: Putting Them All Together, Updated March 27, 2014, Published March 23, 2012 by Jacquie Craig, MS, RD, LD, CDE on https://www.diabetesselfmanagement.com

head around the idea that the most important part of a meal, the one that "fills your stomach", should not be based on cereals or their by-products, but on vegetables and fruit.

- When possible, make "smart" replacements of similar foods, but with lower load. For instance, muesli (GI 57) instead of corn flakes for breakfast (GI 104); rye or buckwheat bread instead of wheat bread (rye flour has a GI of 29 compared to 66 for wheat flour).

- Very important: By correctly combining foods, the overall glycemic index is lowered (and therefore also the load). In the stomach everything is mixed: so foods with many fibers, for instance, slow down the absorption of carbohydrates, as if they were inside the original food. For instance, with a vegetable-based condiment the load of a rice or pasta dish decreases.

- Fats have the same effect: Seasoning with extra virgin olive oil dishes with a high glycemic load, for instance, decreases it. We have already seen that you don't have to be afraid of fats, if taken in the right doses and chosen well.

- Always prefer whole grains: Thanks to the fact that they have not been deprived of their natural fiber content, they have a much lower glycemic load.

- Stay away from sugar and everything that contains it. A cake now and then doesn't hurt but taking sugar every day means hearing the famous old lady at the window screaming like a banshee all the time.

So, what about the statement that cereals and their by-products provide us with long-term energy? We now know that it is the glycemic load that determines: the difference between simple and complex carbohydrates concerns their molecular structure, but our body is very quick to transform one into the other, and in the end, both become sugar. So, a food like white bread has a higher glycemic load than, for instance, maple syrup or fructose.

This is proven by the fact that many studies have not found very different effects in weight loss in diets based on simple or complex carbohydrates, all other things being equal[84].

If we want cereals that really release sugars over a longer period of time and less harmful to our glycemia, we should opt for whole-grain ones.

---

[84] Saris et al. Randomized controlled trial of changes in dietary carbohydrate/fat ratio and simple vs complex carbohydrates on body weight and blood lipids: the CARMEN study. The Carbohydrate Ratio Management in European National diets. Int J Obes Relat Metab Disord. 2000 Oct;24(10):1310-8.

PART THREE

Build a Nutritional Program

11.   The Right Composition of the Diet

"The good is beautiful in that it is governed by the right measure, by the general balance, by the mediumship established by the exact laws of virtue, which is harmony."
Diogenes Laertius

In this part of the book, drawing on the knowledge we have accumulated so far, we will try to answer a simple question: what do we need to eat to stay healthy, have maximum energy and live better? And how to lose weight in a simple and lasting way while achieving all these goals?

More specifically, how should the total amount of food we eat be ideally divided between the different categories of food (meat, vegetables, dairy products, etc.) and between the different types of nutrients? If we start combing through the Internet, or in a bookstore, we'll find hundreds of different answers. Remember what we said in the introduction to this book about the dozens and dozens of different diets that sprout like mushrooms everywhere?

There would be nothing wrong with having all this abundance of literature on the subject, were the advice of one book not radically opposed to that of another. There are those who would want us to eat "a bit of everything", as advised by grandma, those who take a crusade against carbohydrates and flour by-products, and those who swear that by eating only vegetable products you can live up to a hundred years. There is the fashionable food of the moment that will change our lives: turmeric! The acai berries! Ginger! And there is the "bad guy" to point the finger at from time to time: milk, red meat, white bread, egg... Putting all this information together, you could conceive of an ideal diet based on not eating anything, so as not to displease anyone. It is a pity that this is not a very healthy regime.

The enormous confusion on the subject stems from the fact that not even the official medical and scientific positions on nutrition have always been clear and unequivocal. If you have read this book so far, you will remember, for instance, the blunders that official medical science has made with regard to fats.

Unfortunately, however, there is much more to it, and it is necessary to talk about it before attempting to give an answer (as always scientific) to the initial question. If you are a fan of political thrillers, you will love this. Now, we talk about conspiracies made behind closed doors in the palaces of power... and high schoolers who stuff themselves with pizza.

The Invasion of the Pink Slime

- A very well-known soft drink brand is investing millions of dollars in researches that should demonstrate the lack of connection between the increase in refined sugars in the diet and obesity: a nice tall glass of this famous drink would be a snack as healthy as a packet of almonds. The statements have cost lawsuits by non-profit organizations[85], which claim that the studies in question, precisely because they are financed by the multinational, highly underestimate the real effects of sugar on health.

In a television advertising campaign, the multinational company defines the calories of this drink can as "happy calories", and suggests, among other things, to burn them by laughing more during the day. Another expedient used in the interviews, for instance, is to shift the focus to a completely different direction, for instance on the theme of hydration. At this Company, they don't believe in empty calories; they believe in hydration. And they offer this important source of life to consumers (who could have done, perhaps, with a glass of water...)

- In the USA, one of the top food companies sells a product which is essentially slices of industrial cheese. Each slice provides more than half the calories from saturated fats, has a high amount of sodium, and a battalion of chemical additives (sodium phosphate, calcium phosphate, sodium citrate...). Technically, according to American regulations, they cannot even be considered cheese. It's not poison, but neither is it a food to eat every day: it should be something to add to your diet once in a while, if you like, as an exception. Yet, the prestigious Academy of Nutrition and Dietetics has allowed the company to print on the packaging the seal "kids eat right", emblem of its

---

[85] Press Release of the 4th of January 2017 of the Center for Science in the Public Interest

national campaign for healthy eating. How is that possible? Reading the small lines, it turns out that the brand is simply a sponsor of the program: the company says that this does not mean in any way that the association advises to consume it as part of a balanced diet. But how clear is this to consumers, many people wonder[86]? Isn't this some form of corporate prostitution?

- The American Congress has decided that pizza is a vegetable[87]. In school canteens in the United States, meals subsidized by the Federal Government must contain a certain amount of vegetables by law; this is to promote healthy food consumption in kids, and to prevent them from eating fast food, potato chips and nutritionally poor food every day. When the decision was made, the lobby representing the manufacturers of frozen pizza (fearing a decrease in profits) used all their influence in Washington to claim that, from a legal point of view, the tomato sauce contained in a slice of frozen industrial pizza is enough to consider it a vegetable. With all due respect to eggplants and zucchini…

- What's the "pink slime"? It is not the secretion of some B-movie alien, but the colloquial name of an industrial preparation made from offcuts and remainders from the slaughter of meat animals. Cartilage and other processing waste that no one would buy is ground and treated with chemicals until it becomes a bright pink compound. In the United States, the pink slime is used for the preparation of many meat products, to the point of being present in 70% of them. There are several questions, all quite understandable, about the quality of this product. Among the main ones, a request from the U.S. Agricultural Marketing Service to determine the consequences of the presence of ammonia in the dough on the health of consumers, following various protests against the penetrating smell that the slime emanated. A large multinational producer of the slime won the lawsuit that would have forced it to list ammonia among the ingredients, discouraging use and purchase of the slime. Thanks to the support of the meat industry lobby, perhaps, the burgers you have in the fridge have in part the same composition as the solvent in the bathroom[88].

[86] A Cheese 'Product' Gains Kids' Nutrition Seal, By , MARCH 12, 2015 3:28 PM March 12, 2015 3:28 pm 145, New York Times blog

[87] Huffington Post, How Pizza Became A Vegetable Through The Magic Of Influence-Peddling, 11/16/2011 04:20 pm ET | Updated Jan 16, 2012

These few picturesque examples should make you start looking at what you eat with different eyes; however, the mother of all food lobbying operations is much bigger and has had truly devastating effects.

The Cursed Pyramid

From a dietary point of view, the world is in bad health. Very bad, actually. In the United States, more than a third of adults are obese, and almost a fifth of young people and children; the trend of expanding waistline is common to all industrialized countries[89].

Heart disease, in parallel, has become the leading cause of death in the world: one in three people, in practice, goes to a better place for disorders related to the cardiovascular system[90]. Type-two diabetes, the one associated with poor nutrition, is also becoming a real global epidemic, crossing the borders of industrialized countries to touch developing countries as well[91].

These problems have particularly intensified in the past few decades. What has happened? You can certainly point the finger at the opulent society and the increasingly easy availability of junk food, fast food and candies... yet it is quite logical that these factors alone cannot explain such a radical spread of obesity and nutrition-related diseases. There must necessarily be something more radical; on the other hand, it is in common experience to fight against weight or at least to have a flaccid belly already at the age of 40, as well as to feel weak, worn out and without energy, or to undergo an early and dangerous aging of the entire cardiovascular system. What has happened in these last decades? Did some mad scientist fly over our skies spraying some mysterious

---

[88] HUFFINGTON POST, Pink Slime, Ammonium Hydroxide Fast Food Ground Beef Additive, Dropped By McDonald's Et Al., 01/27/2012 04:38 pm ET | **Updated** Mar 05, 2012

[89] Psychiatr Clin North Am. Author manuscript; available in PMC 2012 Dec 1., Published in final edited form as:, Psychiatr Clin North Am. 2011 Dec; 34(4): 717–732., doi: 10.1016/j.psc.2011.08.005, OBESITY: OVERVIEW OF AN EPIDEMIC, Nia Mitchell, MD, Vicki Catenacci, MD, Holly R. Wyatt, MD, and James O. Hill, PhD

[90] World Health Organisation fact sheet, settembre 2016

[91] The New York Times, The Global Diabetes Epidemic, By KASIA LIPSKAAPRIL 25, 2014

poison? None of this; much more simply, we are discovering that "official" advice on how to eat has no scientific basis... Let's try to better understand why.

It is very likely that you have already seen the food pyramid. It is a very simple visual model that should give you a glimpse of what we should eat every day to stay healthy. It was conceived by the U.S. Department of Agriculture in 1992 by re-adapting a Swedish idea from the 1970s. The messages that the 1992 pyramid gives roughly correspond to what most people consider to be "common sense nutrition", and this is proof of how much these indications have pervaded eating habits around the world:

• At the base of the pyramid are the foods that must be most widely consumed, and on which our daily diet must be based: cereals and their by-products. Recommended 6 to 11 servings per day.

• On the upper level, fruit and vegetables, to be consumed in abundance, from 5 to 9 total recommended portions.

• As we move upwards, the pyramid begins to shrink, and we enter the field of foods on which we must pay a little more attention: dairy products (2-3 portions) and animal products such as eggs, meat or fish (2-3 portions).

• In the tip, foods to be consumed only occasionally and with caution: sweets, oils and fats.

IN THE ORIGINAL FOOD PYRAMID, THE CARBOHYDRATE IS THE KING.

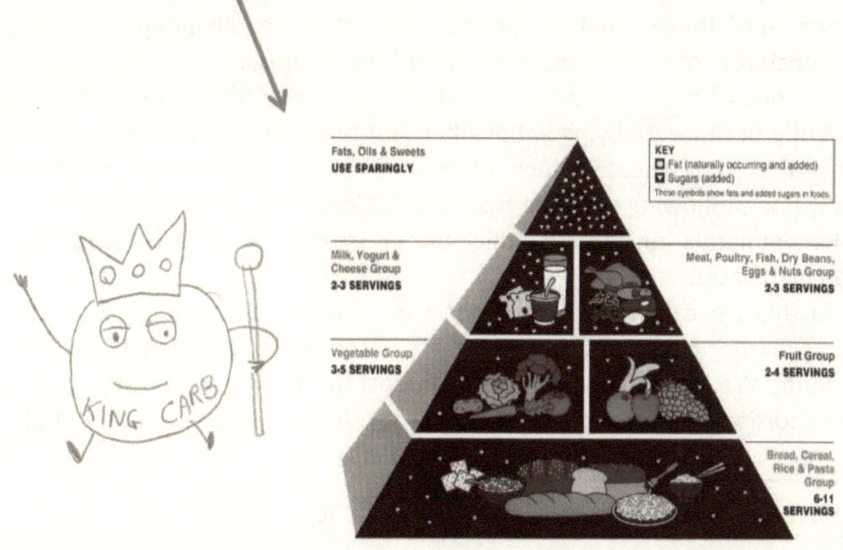

Do you find yourselves in these directions? Do an experiment: share them with ten random people you know. The vast majority, I bet, will consider them totally reasonable. If you remember some of the concepts explained earlier in this book, however, it may be that you now have some doubts.

Luise Light was responsible for the original project for the U.S. government and therefore knows the pyramid very well. In an article from 2004[92] she says verbatim:

"When our version of the Food Guide came back to us revised, we were shocked to find that it was vastly different from the one we had developed. As I later discovered, the wholesale changes made to the guide by the Office of the Secretary of Agriculture were calculated to win the acceptance of the food industry".

What are the changes reported by Luise? Here are the main ones:

To please the farmers in the sector, the portions of cereals had been greatly increased: as we have seen, from 6 to 11 per day (3 or 4 in the original version). Biscuits for breakfast, crackers as a morning snack, pasta for lunch followed by a loaf of bread, crispbread in the afternoon, rice for dinner... does that sound like a lot to you? Yet we are only six portions, the minimum according to the revisited pyramid...

The products derived from refined white flour, moreover, had been expressly indicated as unhealthy and taken to the top of the pyramid. Imagine Luise's expression when she saw them show off in the base of the pyramid, among the things that must be consumed in abundance... lobby of manufacturers of snacks, pop-tarts, bread substitutes...

Portions of fresh fruit and vegetables had been reduced (from 5-9 to 2-3), evidently because lobbying actions had not been strong enough in this regard (growing corn or wheat is much more profitable...). They will be increased to 5-7 only later, following pressure from the National Cancer Institute.

Recommendations to generally prefer fresh food to processed one had been eliminated.

To this we can add, even if not expressly mentioned in the article, the discriminatory treatment given to fats: relegated as lepers at the top of the pyramid. We already know that, except for hydrogenated fats or those disproportionate in omega six, they do not deserve this reputation at all, and

---

[92] A Fatally Flawed Food Guide, by Luise Light, Ed.D, 2004

that a generous pour of extra virgin olive oil on our salad is only beneficial for us.

"I vehemently protested that the changes, if followed, could lead to an epidemic of obesity and diabetes - and couldn't be justified on either health or nutritional grounds. To my amazement, I was a lone voice on this issue, as my colleagues appeared to accept the 'policy level' decision."

Real Cassandra of the nutrition, Luise had, as you can see, predicted right. The guidelines changed the traditional common sense, making absolutely natural foods (meat, cheese, olive oil...) perceived as dangerous and replacing them with industrial products rich in refined flours and sugar, cheap to produce, which brought enormous profits to the food industries.

Not only that: the "low fat" industry, in this wake, has become a huge business; too bad that fat has been replaced in packaged foods, once again, by carbohydrates.

Between recommendations and proliferation of packaged products on the shelves, carbohydrates have taken control over our diet.

"It is true: the focus on fat reduction in the recommended daily doses has implicitly led to an increase in carbohydrates," says Dr. Walter Willett, head of the Department of Nutrition at Harvard's School of Public Health. "And this has become problematic, because the vast majority of carbohydrates in the United States are refined and bad for health"[93].

We have already seen how refined carbohydrates are very closely related to diabetes, obesity and heart disease, so we should not be surprised if the incidence rates of these problems have exploded in parallel with the transposition of these guidelines.

To dispel any doubt about this, we quote a study from 2004[94] that analyzes the statistical correlation between type-two diabetes and consumption of refined carbohydrates in the United States during the twentieth century and that confirms, without a shadow of a doubt, the relationship between the two variables.

---

[93] Huffington Pot, What The Government Got Wrong About Nutrition — And How It Can Fix It, By Meredith Melnick, Sabrina Siddiqui, 31/7/2014

[94] © 2004 American Society for Clinical Nutrition, Increased consumption of refined carbohydrates and the epidemic of type 2 diabetes in the United States: an ecologic assessment, Lee S Gross, , Li Li, , Earl S Ford, and Simin Liu

The Ideal Dish

In 2011, the pyramid was officially retired by the Department of Agriculture and replaced in the official guides for the population by Myplate: the image of a dish divided into parts represents the ideal distribution of a meal. From the point of view of effectiveness and usability, the new version is certainly better. Instead of representing the totality of the food to be eaten during the day and relying on generic and subjective "portions", it offers a visual and simple idea of how, more or less, to extricate oneself between the various foods at each meal. We also have a clear nutritional improvement: the avalanche of carbohydrates is reduced: according to the new guidelines, cereals should occupy about a quarter of the ideal dish, with foods rich in protein that fill it for another quarter and fruit and vegetables for the rest. Dairy products appear as a sort of accompaniment, to the side, in the form of an imaginary glass of milk.

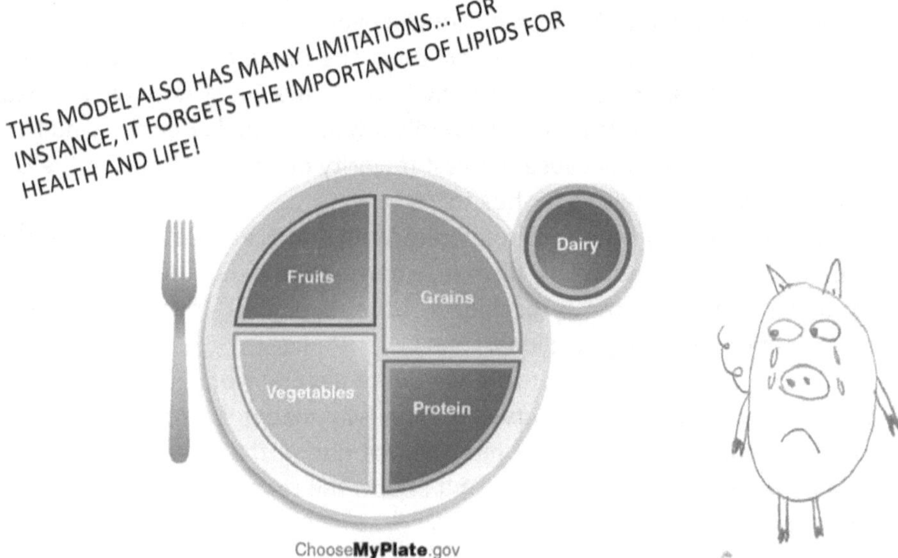

ChooseMyPlate.gov

However, the new scheme still has many limitations, which keep it away from the real ideal diet. These problems have been publicly highlighted by Harvard Medical School, which has prepared an improved version of Myplate called Healthy Living Plate, specifying on their website: "The Healthy Eating Plate is based exclusively on the best available science and was not subjected to political or commercial pressures from food industry lobbyists."

Which sounds like a not-so-veiled accusation against the official work of the government... [95]

What are Harvard's criticisms of Myplate, and what are the consequent changes to improve it?

•   Initially, Myplate did not differentiate between refined and whole grains. Later, the advice to consume at least half of the daily cereals in the form of whole grains was added, but this is still not enough ... the Harvard model expressly encourages to limit as much as possible refined grains, crowning whole grains as the main choice

•   Myplate is silent about the fats chapter. Looking at the representation of the dish, you might think that it is right to completely eliminate fats. We have already talked many times about their absolute necessity for health. Harvard's plate, on the other hand, has a small bottle of oil drawn to the side to remember the central role of these substances, and then rightly details which to prefer, in line with what we have already seen

•   Harvard recommends drinking water at every meal, limiting fruit juices as much as possible (rich in sugar and poor in nutrients; Myplate instead considers them as portions of fruit if 100%) and reducing milk and dairy products to two portions a day (dairy products are not a necessary accompaniment to every meal as Myplate seems to communicate)

Let's go back to our initial question: what do you need to eat to stay healthy, have maximum energy and live better? It is likely that the Harvard model is a very good answer, which is easy to prove when you consider that it is in accordance with everything we have seen together so far.

Below is the detail of the Healthy Eating Plate recommendations:

---

[95] https://www.hsph.harvard.edu/nutritionsource/healthy-eating-plate-vs-usda-myplate/

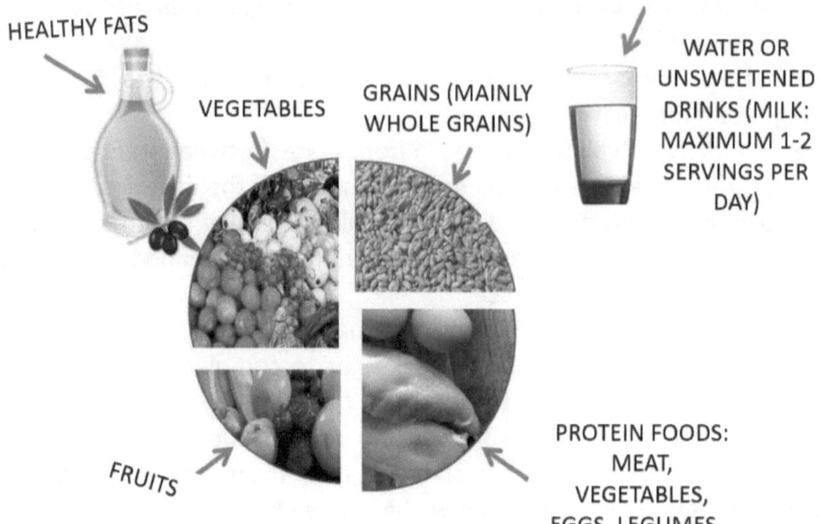

Thinking of an ideal plate containing one of our meals, half should be filled with fresh fruit and vegetables; the vegetables should fill two thirds of this half and the fruit the rest. The variety is very important, better to change often types of vegetables. Beware of potatoes, which count as bread, not as vegetables.

A quarter of the total plate must be filled with cereals and their by-products, which must be whole-grain. Refined cereals and their by-products, on the other hand, should only be consumed occasionally, as an exception.

The other quarter should be filled with protein-rich foods, such as white meats, fish, legumes, eggs and (in more moderation) red meats and cheeses. Processed meats, on the other hand, should be eaten occasionally.

It is important not to forget to season with healthy oils (such as extra virgin olive oil and canola oil, but you could add to the list of healthy fats also fatty fish, avocado, oilseeds, dried fruit). Butter should be consumed in more moderation, and trans fats should be avoided altogether.

It is also important to drink water or sugar-free alternatives (tea, coffee). Milk and dairy products are not a substitute for water, but a real food to be consumed at most once or twice a day, while sugary drinks, including fruit juices, should be avoided.

This model is effective precisely because it is very simple. It allows you not to get lost in abstruse classifications or strict rules, but to have an effective idea of how daily food should be distributed. It is obvious that it is not always possible to distribute every meal in this way, but it is useful to have this graphic representation in front of our eyes so that, during the course of the day, what we eat represents, more or less, the various groups of foods in these proportions.

There is no need to become obsessed with this: perhaps the deficiencies of one day can be recovered in the next, the important thing is that there is harmony between the various categories. As you can see, it's not anything dramatic or disruptive; it's simply the obvious consequence of how our body's biochemistry works.

Sweets, fried and packaged foods are not mentioned and therefore, along with refined grains and processed meats, should be considered an exception. There is nothing wrong with eating them once or twice a week, perhaps on weekends; the important thing is that they are not made absolutely the basis of nutrition.

These rules for the "ideal dish" also allow, as is easy to verify, to comply with the instructions we have given previously to keep under control the glycemic load: from wherever you get there, good food is good food.

12. Calories and Body Weight

" Animals fill themselves; man eats. The man of mind alone knows how to eat"
Jean Anthelme Brillat-Savarin

Lulu's Obsession

We have understood how our diet must be structured so that we can live well, for a long time and full of energy. The next question is: how do we have to behave in order to lose (or gain) weight?

This is no small question, given the multimillion-dollar, and never-in-crisis, business that concerns books, medicines, supplements, courses and special foods aimed at weight loss. Once again, we want to tackle this issue from a scientific point of view, without being influenced by current fashions and the endless pseudo-scientific literature on the subject.

Body fat, as we have previously seen in detail, is nothing more than an energy store: the excess nutrients introduced with the food end up there to be burned in lean times. It is a mechanism that allowed us to survive when we were cave dwellers who could find food every other day; but today, in the age of snack vending machines, it has backfired against us.

It is precisely in terms of energy that we must therefore think. The main measure of the energy that food provides is borrowed from thermodynamics, and you all certainly know it very well: the calorie.

A calorie (or, more properly, a kilocalorie, even if in this case we will use the first, more common term for simplicity), is nothing but a quantity of energy.

More precisely, the one necessary to raise by one degree centigrade the temperature of one kilo of distilled water at the pressure of an atmosphere.

So, when we eat a 500-calorie chocolate bar, we provide our mitochondria with enough fuel to produce the same amount of energy that would raise by one degree the temperature of more than 1.000 pounds of water... be honest, you didn't think you were small thermostats.

All energy-consuming activities are also measured in calories, with the same logic.

The first person in history to spread the idea of using calorie counts for weight loss to the public was Dr. Lulu Hunt Peters. Back in 1918, she was a pioneer in dietetics, and churned out the first bestseller on weight loss in history: *Diet and health*[96].

Born in Maine and moved to California as a young woman, Lulu had always been overweight: she had weighed almost 220 pounds. After graduating in medicine from Berkeley in 1909, Lulu decided to apply her medical knowledge to the connection between calories and weight loss. Not only did she manage to lose nearly 70 pounds of weight, but she also devoted herself completely to the subject, launching a public awareness campaign on the themes of weight control, exercise and diet.

Nowadays, many parts of this book will naturally bring a smile to your face: for instance, those warning against the trends of the time to lose weight, which included pills based on arsenic, or even pills containing larvae of intestinal parasites...

Moreover, the approach to weight loss is certainly not that of a rational doctor... Lulu seemed mostly obsessed with the subject, as testified by these two passages of her book, which we report as evidence of how much the

---

[96] *Jou, Chin (2007-10-11). "Your Stomach Must Be Disciplined": Lulu Hunt Peters and the Beginnings of Calorie-Counting in Corporeal Self-Regulation, 1918-1924. Annual Meeting of The American Studies Association. Philadelphia Marriott Downtown, Philadelphia, PA. Retrieved 17 October 2013.*

culture on the subject has changed (fortunately). Between ill-concealed contempt for anyone who doesn't want to be a skeleton, manipulative husbands and friends with macabre stories, we have quite an interesting sample of the neuroses of the beginning of the twentieth century...

"Are You Thin and Do You Want to Gain? Skip this chapter. It will not interest you in the least. I will come to you later. I am not particularly interested in you anyway, for I cannot get your point of view. How anyone can want to be anything but thin is beyond my intelligence. However, knowing that there are such deluded individuals, I have been constrained to give you advice..."

"When you start to reduce you will have the following to combat. First: Your husband, who tells you that he does not like thin women. I almost hate my husband when I think how long he kept me under that delusion. Now, of course, I know all about his jealous disposition, and how he did not want me to be attractive. Second: Your sister, who says, "Goodness, Lou, but you look old today; you looked lots better as you were! Third: Your friends, who tell you that you are just right now; don't lose another pound! And other friends who tell you cheerful tales of people they have known who reduced, and who went into a decline, and finally died"[97].

Despite these aspects, however balanced by the delightful illustrations made by Lulu's 9-year-old nephew (some of which deserve to be seen, we bring them back in these pages!), the core message of the book is incredibly topical.

---

[97] "Diet and health", 1918, Lulu Hunt Peters

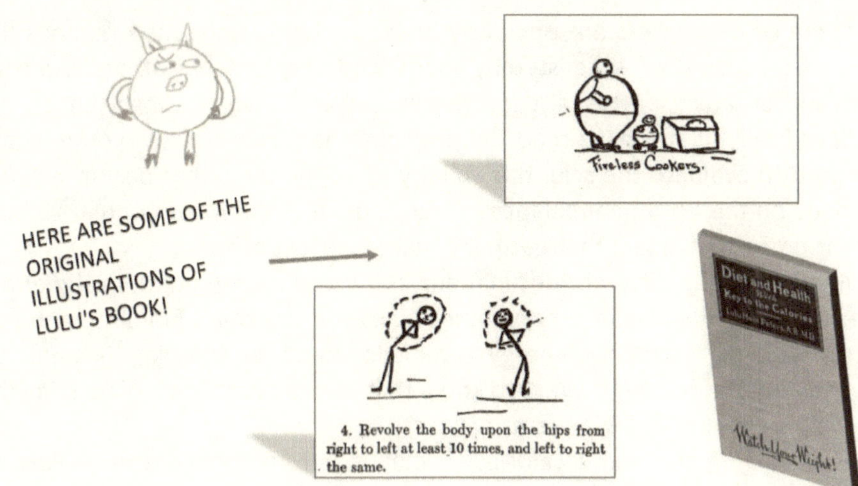

Quite simply, Lulu claimed that the key to losing weight was to ingest less calories than were consumed. That's it. The book then made it possible to calculate the daily calorie requirement on the basis of parameters such as gender, height, physical activity ... and estimate the amount of calories of the various foods.

This simple truth underlies all the diets that came later, and it is still the official point of view of medicine. The diets that any doctor will make you are calculated just as Lulu would have done:

- estimation of your individual daily caloric requirement, which also takes into account your physical activity.

- reduction of the same by an acceptable percentage, which corresponds to the calories that your body will take from adipose tissue instead of food.

- distribution of the calories left on your daily menu.

However, many theories, more or less recent, do not agree with this simple way of proceeding. "Not all calories are equal!", is the mantra of these diets. The dissertations that motivate them are diverse, but they all have in common the attempt to try to circumvent the hard law of "eat less, move more": therefore, there would be special combinations of food that allow a faster weight loss. The offers are almost endless and for all tastes: diets without carbohydrates, without meat, without grains, with only vegetables, without dairy products, with specific percentages of the different nutrients...

Some of these diets are obviously hoax, or clearly unhealthy regimes (like the classic "soup diet" suggested by your friend's cousin), but others also come from authoritative sources, and it is therefore worth investigating them.

Specifically, if you have read the previous chapters carefully, you might be tempted to evaluate the scientific validity of all the diets that base the choice of foods on the hormonal balance of our body. It is the most popular trend in recent times, and in fact the reasoning makes perfect sense.

Apart from the different declinations and theories, the point, in the end, is this: we know that insulin, among other functions, has that of inhibiting the use of our adipose tissue for energy production, and to stimulate instead the accumulation of body fat. We also know that carbohydrate-rich diets stimulate insulin production, so logic seems flawless:

"Considering the same calories, a diet rich in carbohydrates makes me produce more insulin, thus accumulating more fat and burning less."

"Conversely, given the same number of calories, a diet poor in carbohydrates makes me produce less insulin, thus accumulating less fat and burning more".

Hence the famous motto that "not all calories are equal": if the above statements are true, eating a thousand calories of dried beef is not the same as eating as many calories of bread. The common denominator of this new line of diets, in fact, is the famous "low carb" trend.

It is, however, a useless extreme. On the one hand, it is true that it is necessary to keep insulin under control, as we have widely shown, to gain health and to avoid entering the vicious circle of insulin resistance, which in fact makes us accumulate fat more easily.

If, however, you remain in an acceptable window of glycemic index and correct mix of foods and nutrients, it is completely unnecessary to fear carbohydrates and avoid them like the plague.

Do you want some proof?

The Junk Food Diet

Writer Jeff Wilser has tested himself on a very odd diet: nothing but junk food for a month: cookies, candies, chocolate, fries... everything a person on a diet keeps themselves well away from. No fruit, no vegetables, no healthy food. With one important limitation, however: count all the calories and do not exceed a set quantity.

By the end of the month, Jeff had lost almost 11 pounds. So much so that his doctor said that "one should not lose so much weight in such a short time". Even all his blood values had no particular issues[98].

Before you all decide to convert to a diet of tacos and pancakes, it is necessary to make two important points. First, the nutrient mix is important for your health in the long term. If you prolong such a diet over time, you run the risk of serious problems, which you can easily imagine if you have carefully read the previous chapters: a real self-destruction of your body.

This experiment makes us understand that it is the balance between ingested and consumed calories that makes us lose or gain weight. The food mix is very important, but it's more about our health. Therefore, eating healthy food remains essential, unless you want to be the thinnest in the cemetery. But the crusades against carbohydrates make no sense, and treating ourselves to a fragrant sandwich, or a plate of pasta will not compromise our diet. Just as, once in a while, indulging in a little treat... in the end, food must be a pleasure, right?

A second consideration to make: Jeff was evidently in good health when he started this bizarre diet. In particular, his insulin cycle was normal, so he could well absorb the temporary mega-surplus of blood sugars. The other dark side of this type of nutrition, is in fact, as you know, the risk of insulin resistance... with all the dangers it brings.

If your metabolism is already compromised by excess sugars, refined carbohydrates and other hyper-insulinizing foods, Jeff's diet probably would not make you lose weight. Instead, in this case, it would be advisable to "reset" the insulin cycle with at least one month of low-glycemic diet (if you want to

---

[98] The Good News About What's Bad for You (and Vice Versa) *by Jeff Wilser*, Affirm Press, January 2016

try it, just choose the low-load foods in the list, always keeping an eye on the correct mix of foods).

Taking into consideration everything we have seen so far, you have at this point a logical path to follow:

• determine the individual caloric requirement, net of any physical activity.

• reduce it by the amount necessary for a gradual loss of weight.

• "spread" the resulting calories on a variety of foods that respects the breakdowns of the Harvard model. In doing so, try to focus on the variety, so that most of the diet is composed of natural foods (see what we said in "Let's take a first stock of the situation").

• If you wish, you can "adjust" any of the meals by including what you like, no matter what... as long as the calorie count is respected in these meals too. In addition, add one "free" meal per week without any problems

Here is the procedure for building a diet that is healthy, scientifically proven, effective, and flexible enough to allow us to enjoy life. In the rest of the book, we will guide you step by step through the process of building it, keeping in mind that it can be customized according to one's needs, thus not only for those who want to lose weight, but also for those who just need to maintain it or, with all due respect to Lulu, must gain it.

Before starting this process, however, just as we have done so far, we want to give a solid scientific basis to the observations made. In particular, we want to disprove those studies bearing witness to the slimming effects of "low carb" diets which seem to contradict the simple mathematics of calories.

As Michael Matthews explains very effectively in his book, *Bigger, leaner, stronger,* quite simply, the diets low in carbohydrates that are proposed in these studies are usually very rich in protein. Proteins, as we know, are a fundamental component of our muscle mass, and in fact one of the main risks of an unbalanced restrictive diet is to lose lean mass instead of adipose tissue. If on the other hand, the protein intake during a diet is higher than normal, the muscle mass is preserved, and this in turn helps weight loss in various ways. As a matter of fact, muscle cells need more energy than adipose tissue cells to function[99].

---

[99] Bigger Leaner Stronger: The Simple Science of Building the Ultimate Male Body, Michael Matthews, Oculus Publishers, 2012

On the other hand, the diets with more carbohydrates with which the comparison is made are also low in protein. So, this is what happens:

- Many carbohydrates and few proteins -> loss of muscle mass -> slowing down of metabolism -> much less effective weight loss
- Few carbohydrates and many proteins -> maintenance or increase of muscle mass -> acceleration of metabolism -> more effective weight loss

To test this theory, it would then be necessary to compare two high carb/low carb diets with the same amount of protein, and calories.

Michael Matthews reports several studies with these characteristics, and the result confirms the assumption: if you prevent the loss of lean mass, low carb diets are, for equal calories, as effective as high carb ones[100]. Therefore, the important thing is, with all the due clarifications mentioned above, the balance between energy introduced and energy consumed. The good old Lulu, despite everything, still wins.

Living on Air

Speaking of bizarre theories about food, here's something that beats them all. Do you know about breatharianism? It is a theory (we swear, it really exists) according to which it is possible to survive without eating, drawing one's nourishment from the breath, absorbing the energy of the universe (or of the sun, it seems). It seems impossible, but there are people who support this theory.

In 1999, the Australian breatharian Ellen Greve, who claimed she hadn't eaten or drunk anything for over five years, agreed to participate in a sort of television experiment. She was filmed for a week, all the time, to show that she was surviving without introducing any liquids or solids into her body. Already on the second day, she showed worrying symptoms of dehydration. Ellen claimed that air pollution was interfering with the purity of the energy she breathed, and was transferred to the mountains. Here too, however,

---

[100] © 2006 American Society for Clinical Nutrition, Ketogenic low-carbohydrate diets have no metabolic advantage over nonketogenic low-carbohydrate diets, Carol S Johnston, , Sherrie L Tjonn, , Pamela D Swan, Andrea White, Heather Hutchins, and Barry Sears

dehydration issues continued, and were soon accompanied by weight loss and even trouble talking. The program was interrupted[101].

With all due respect to the breatharians, it is therefore established that, whether we like it or not, we must consume calories throughout the day. This is also, as we have seen, the first step towards making a tailor-made and scientifically proven diet.

The calories we need during the day are given by the sum of the basal and kinetic metabolic rate. The basal metabolic rate is nothing more than the amount of calories that we need for the normal functioning of our body at rest: to make the heart beat, to make us breathe, to make all organs and cells work. The kinetic requirement must be added to it, i.e. the energy needed for each type of physical activity (not only sports, but also any movement we do: getting up, walking, etc.).

To calculate the Basal Metabolic Rate (BMR), we will use the Harris-Benedict formula[102], conceived for the first time at the beginning of the century, and later revisited in a study in 1990[103]. The formula estimates how many calories a person needs to rest based on age, height and weight. It is the most widely used in the technical field.

You can find it below in two versions: with centimeters / kilograms and with pounds / inches

Metric formula for men
BMR = (10 × weight in kg) + (6.25 × height in cm) – (5 × age in years) + 5

Imperial formula for men
BMR = (4.536 × weight in pounds) + (15.88 × height in inches) – (5 × age) + 5

Metric formula for women
BMR = (10 × weight in kg) + (6.25 × height in cm) – (5 × age in years) – 161

---

[101] http://news.bbc.co.uk/2/hi/uk_news/scotland/453661.stm

[102] Harris JA, Benedict FG (1918). "A Biometric Study of Human Basal Metabolism". Proceedings of the National Academy of Sciences of the United States of America. 4 (12): 370–3. doi:10.1073/pnas.4.12.370. PMC 1091498. PMID 16576330.

[103] Mifflin MD, St Jeor ST, Hill LA, Scott BJ, Daugherty SA, Koh YO (1990). "A new predictive equation for resting energy expenditure in healthy individuals". *The American Journal of Clinical Nutrition*. 51 (2): 241–7. PMID 2305711

Imperial formula for women

BMR = (4.536 × weight in pounds) + (15.88 × height in inches) – (5 × age) – 161

The kinetic requirement must then be added to the basal metabolic rate. The kinetic requirement is estimated by multiplying the basal metabolic rate by an index that depends on the level of average daily activity:

No physical activity, sedentary lifestyle = 1.2

Light physical activity = 1.375

Moderate physical activity = 1.55

Heavy physical activity = 1.725

Very heavy physical activity= 1.9

To give you a more precise idea of these indexes:

- A person who practices an amateur sport, or trains in the gym, less than three times a week and always walks at least a little during the day is in the "light" category.
- A person who practices an amateur sport, or trains in the gym at least three times a week, always walks at least a little during the day and has a sedentary job is in the "moderate" category.

Not many people can be considered to be in the "heavy" category. This is, for instance, the case for people who train at least three times a week and have in addition a job that involves physical activity

Even fewer people can be counted among those doing "very heavy" activities: professional sportsmen who train every day, or people with hard work. This is because it is quite easy to overestimate our own activities and therefore our own calorie requirements. If you are undecided between two indexes, the advice is to choose the lowest one anyway.

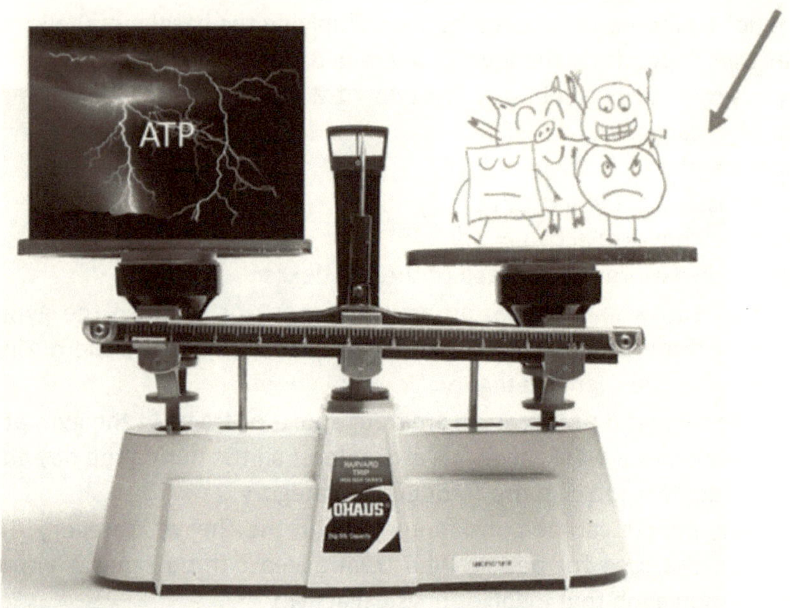

We will give a couple of examples of calculation:

John is a 39-year-old man, 71.7 inches tall and weighs 192 pounds. He plays basketball with his friends once a week, and otherwise does a desk job.

BMR = (4.536 × 192) + (15.88 × 71.7) − (5 × 39) + 5 = 1,818 calories

To obtain the daily requirement we must multiply this by the index reflecting the kinetic requirement. In this case the activity level is sedentary, so the daily requirement is equal to 1,818 X 1.2 = 2,182 calories.

Kate is a 25-year-old woman, 66.1 inches tall and weighs 132 pounds. She trains in the gym three times a week, and in addition she has a very active lifestyle: she is always on the move during the day, she has a dynamic job, she walks a lot...

BMR = (4.536 × 132) + (15.88 × 66.1) − (5 × 25) − 161 = 1,364 calories

To obtain the daily requirement we must multiply this by the index reflecting the kinetic requirement. In this case the activity level is moderate, so the daily requirement is equal to 1,364 X 1.55 = 2,114 calories.

The next step in preparing a diet for weight loss is, at this point, to subtract from the total calories thus obtained the part that, every day, should not come from food, but from the fat that we already have inside. The question at this point is simple: how much should this part be?

The best answer must necessarily depend on a percentage of your daily needs, and not on a fixed number. The reason is simple: in this way people who have a greater need for energy (taking into account the factors considered above, therefore physical characteristics and daily activities) will have the opportunity to eat, in proportion, more. On the other hand, people with a lower need will have a calorie deficit more appropriate to their constitution and/or lifestyle.

For this purpose, we set three reduction percentages for the daily requirement:

Low: -15%

Average: -20%

High: -25%

Which one's better? The answer is quite an individual one: it's like asking someone if they prefer to step into the cold water of a swimming pool gradually or with a dive. But choosing the percentage that suits you gives you a lot more chance of success. Here are a few points to consider when making your decision:

•   Speed of weight loss: It is clear that the higher the percentage, the faster you lose weight. In addition, high percentages make it lose proportionally more than low percentages. If you prefer to make greater sacrifices for a shorter time and think that your willpower works better this way, go with a high percentage[104].

•   Daily management: On the other hand, the lower the percentage, the more manageable the daily diet. For some people, it's more motivating to lose weight quickly[105]; for others, it's more motivating to have a regime that doesn't make them feel so hungry. If you are in between, you can opt for the average percentage.

---

[104] Saris WH. Very-low-calorie diets and sustained weight loss. *Obes Res.* 2001;9 Suppl 4:295S–301S. doi:10.1038/oby.2001.134.

[105] Astrup A, Rossner S. Lessons from obesity management programmes: greater initial weight loss improves long-term maintenance. *Obes Rev.* 2000;1(1):17–19. Available at: http://www.ysonut.fr/pdf/Ysodoc/C0702.pdf.

- Physical activity: If your daily requirement is calculated taking into account important physical activities (for sport or work), you should probably choose a low percentage, so as to compromise them as little as possible[106].

- Impact on your body and metabolism: If you are generally not in good shape, it is better to start with low deficits. Always remember to consult a specialist before embarking on any dietary regimen.

With reference to the examples we have given, let's suppose that John opts for an average deficit and Kate for a low one.

Their correct caloric requirement for the diet would therefore be:

For John, 2,182 x (1-20%) = 1,745

For Kate, 2,114 x (1-15%) = 1,796

All this is conceived in the case of a diet aimed at weight loss. It goes without saying that the same reasoning can be done if it is necessary to gain weight (by adding the different percentages instead of removing them), and that instead the caloric requirement should be left unchanged if you simply want to preserve your weight by eating as healthy as possible.

A Tailor-Made Diet

And here we are at the last stage of the process: "spreading" the daily calories on the foods to be consumed during the day. As a guide for the calorie content of the main foods, you can refer to Appendix E (be careful: the values refer to 100 grams, or 3.5 ounces, of each food). The table obviously does not claim to be exhaustive: for foods that do not appear on it, a search on the Internet can help you; for packaged foods, you can also refer to the table of nutritional values.

Using these values, you can draft your own diet that "focuses" on the calories you need to reach every day, thus making it fit your tastes and lifestyle. Also, you can plan different alternatives for different days of the week.

It remains to be understood, however, how to distribute the calories throughout the day, and between the various categories of food. We don't want all the daily needs to come from chocolate eaten in the evening, do we?

---

[106] Rodriguez NR, Di Marco NM, Langley S. American College of Sports Medicine position stand. Nutrition and athletic performance. *Med Sci Sports Exerc*. 2009;41(3):709–731.

This calculation could be handled in an extremely complicated way, with recommended percentages of distribution of calories between the various meals, and of distribution between the various macronutrients ... but we believe that if we keep things simple, it is easier to stick to them. It is therefore better to have a few, simple and flexible rules.

As for the distribution between meals, simply choose the one that suits your lifestyle best. It is not true that breakfast must necessarily be abundant[107]: it is another of the food myths imposed on us by the lobbies. Of course, eating in the morning helps you not to feel hungry during the day, but if you feel good with a light breakfast, don't worry. The important thing is the total calories of the day; you decide whether to divide them into many snacks or three main meals. Rely on what makes you feel best about your digestive and energy levels, and your daily needs in terms of time and effort. The more your diet is set up according to your well-being and your real needs, the more pleasant and easy it will be to follow!

On the subject of the distribution between the various types of foods and macronutrients, we believe that the simplest and most effective way is to refer to the Harvard dish we discussed above. This, as we said, to avoid going crazy with obsessive and useless breakdowns that turn the diet into a cage. Simply, when drafting your diet, imagine that everything you eat during the day ends up in a big dish, and do everything you can to respect the distribution we have talked about.

Go back and read the chapter "Let's Take a First Stock of the Situation" for a guide on the foods closest to their natural state (in doing so you will also automatically be more confident about the glycemic load). Make sure that the vast majority of what you eat comes from this type of food, whenever possible. The above considerations should allow you, on the other hand, to have sufficient flexibility to handle special meals of all kinds (at the airport, at the restaurant, at a party ...)

Make sure you vary your food as much as possible! Have fun exploring new fresh foods: fruits, vegetables or cereals other than those you normally eat, new recipes for meat or fish... This is to avoid that the diet becomes a monotonous sadness based on chicken breasts and salad every single day, but also to ensure the full spectrum of nutrients that your body needs... By

[107] Critical Reviews in Food Science and Nutrition , Volume 50, 2010 - Issue 2, Systematic Review Demonstrating that Breakfast Consumption Influences Body Weight Outcomes in Children and Adolescents in Europe, Hania Szajewska & Marek Ruszczyński

rereading the first chapters, you should get a fairly accurate idea of the importance of this aspect.

On the subject of "cheats" and "free meals": food is first of all pleasure. Some foods are real nutritional junk, but we should try not to obsess over nutrition. If you want to, you won't die for cheating once in a while. A good compromise to avoid ruining your diet without having the feeling of living in deprivation could be the following:

Have every week a "day of rebellion against Harvard" and a "meal of total rebellion". On the "day of rebellion against Harvard", you reach your daily calories irrespective of the rule of food distribution... eat what you want and when you want, just do not exceed the recommended calories. In the "meal of total rebellion" (to be done in addition, on another day), treat yourself to what you want, without rules. Obviously, with a bit of common sense: you don't have to eat forcedly, compulsively or until you feel sick, just treat yourself to something you feel like without a thought. This is just an idea, which could be a good compromise. It may also be, and we hope, that your body, purified of industrial and refined foods, will no longer feel the need for such "cheats" ....

Here, by way of example, is a possible day of John's diet.

Breakfast:
200 grams/7 ounces of natural yoghurt: 92 calories
30 grams/1 ounce of wholemeal bread: 60 calories
15 grams/0.5 ounce of walnuts: 100 calories

Snack:
200 grams/7 ounces of apple: 108 calories

Lunch:
100 grams/3.5 ounces of brown rice: 116 calories
10 grams/0.4 ounce of parmesan cheese: 39 calories
220 grams/7.8 ounces of veal chop: 246 calories
200 grams/7 ounces of fresh spinach: 30 calories
25 grams/0.9 ounce of wholemeal bread: 50 calories
25 grams/0.9 ounce of extra virgin olive oil: 225 calories
100 grams/3.5 ounces of pineapple: 57 calories

Snack:
200 grams/7 ounces of strawberries: 66 calories

Dinner:
150 grams/5.3 ounces of eggs: 239 calories
200 grams/7 ounces of tomatoes: 34 calories
155 grams/5.5 ounces of green beans: 54 calories
25 grams/0.9 ounce of wholemeal bread: 50 calories
20 grams/0.7 ounce of extra virgin olive oil: 180 calories

Daily total: 1,746 calories.

PART FOUR

What We Don't Digest

13. What We Don't Digest: Water, Fibers and Life in the Intestine

"If I fight with dung, it is certain that, winner or loser, I will always end up dirtied".
Giacomo Casanova

The Brine of Astronauts

As you can easily imagine, providing the International Space Station with water from Earth is neither easy nor economical (the estimate is about 20,000 $ per gallon...). For this reason, on board everything is programmed not to waste a single drop of water, and especially to recover and recycle everything possible. The oldest system on the ship was developed by the Russians: It purifies and filters the water vapor of breath and sweat, as well as the water used for washing: everything is transformed back into liquid to drink. The new American system goes further: It recycles urine (from humans and even guinea pigs!) and transforms it back into drinking water. Commander Chris Hadfield said that over 90% of the water used comes from these processes... and that it is purer than the water we buy at the supermarket.

The Italian astronaut Samanta Cristoforetti tells, in her logbook[108], how (to use the astronauts' jargon) "to turn yesterday's coffee into tomorrow's coffee". Urine is separated into two products: one is the basis for the new drinking water; the other (which astronauts call "brine" in jargon) contains all the body's waste and is released into space.

The astronaut specifies that she understands how all this can at first seem disturbing or even disgusting. Actually, she continues, if we think of planet

---

[108] http://avamposto42.esa.int/blog/diario-di-bordo/single/l15-trasformare-il-caffe-di-oggi-nel-caffe-di-domani/

Earth as a giant spaceship floating in space, we have to admit that inside it the process is exactly the same: the water molecules are continuously recycled, and the pee of our dog today could be in the very expensive bottle of French mineral water of tomorrow.

Water is essential for life and, without it, human beings can only survive a few days. Our body is made up of water for a percentage of weight ranging from 75% (infants) to 55% (elderly).

Every day we lose part of this amount of water through urine, perspiration and other body fluids, and it is therefore necessary to replace it. Part of this amount (about 20%) is taken through the water contained in food; the rest must necessarily be taken by drinking water or other liquids.

How much though? The Institute of Medicine[109] recommends that men drink at least 101 ounces of water per day, which is a little under 13 cups. Women should drink at least 74 ounces, which is a little over 9 cups. It is important to try to take this amount of water during the day, and not only when you are thirsty (thirst is a kind of "final warning bell" of the body). In addition to water, for instance, squeezed juices, herbal teas, tea, etc. can be taken. These quantities naturally refer to "normal" situations: if, for instance, the physical activity or the external temperature increases, the need increases correspondingly.

Many of the molecules we have encountered in this book undergo various transformations within our bodies: they are disassembled, reassembled and transformed, and from these processes originates the energy that keeps us alive and the same substances that compose us. Water, on the other hand, remains unchanged. Our organism never "breaks" the molecule of water; it does not bind it to anything else: it simply makes it pass through. Why, then, is this substance so indispensable to life that it forces space travelers to extract it from their own pee?

- Water is essential for controlling body temperature. Basically, when we sweat, we expel hot water and, in this way, we lower the temperature of our body within acceptable limits. A hard-working adult can sweat up to around 4 gallons (15 liters) a day. This varies depending on the humidity and the temperature, but even in normal circumstances, the average person sweats up to 1.5 gallons (6 liters) per day. [110].

---

[109] Dietary reference intakes for water, potassium, sodium, chloride and sulfate. Institute of Medicine. http://www.nal.usda.gov/fnic/DRI//DRI_Water/73-185.pdf. Accessed Aug. 12, 2014.

• Water is the main component of blood and plasma, the two liquids carrying around the body the red blood cells that supply us with oxygen, nutrients, hormones... The relationship between the corpuscular part (everything that is not water) and the water in the blood is called hematocrit. If the liquid part decreases too much in relation to the total, the hematocrit increases and the blood, which has become denser, struggles to perform its task, with severe consequences that can also lead to a state of shock.

• Water is also the fundamental component of urine, which purifies the body of harmful substances that would otherwise accumulate in the tissues.

For these reasons, dehydration has grave consequences for the body: It ranges from weakness and dizziness to drowsiness, palpitations, cognitive deficits, hypotension and anxiety. When the volume of blood in circulation decreases to less than about one gallon, the result is loss of consciousness and ultimately death[111].

It is not always enough to drink when you are thirsty, because the stimulus may occur too late. It's much better to keep a bottle of water with you and stay hydrated throughout the day.

Burkitt, the Fiber, and the Secret Position

During World War II, Irish physician Denis Burkitt, while serving with the Royal Army Medical Corps in Kenya and Somalia, noticed how the incidence of colon cancer was much lower among locals than among Europeans. Burkitt came up with two theories to explain this difference.

The first of these has survived to the present day and has brightened up a component of food until then considered only a waste: the dietary fiber[112]. The second one was definitely a bit more awkward, and we will see it at the end of the paragraph...

---

[110] Sawka MN, Latzka WA, Matott RP, Montain SJ. Hydration effects on temperature regulation. Int J Sports Med. 1998;19 (Suppl 2):S108–110 and Sawka MN, Cheuvront SN, Carter R., 3rd Human water needs. Nutr Rev. 2005;63:S30–39.

[111] Mange K; Matsuura D; Cizman B; et al. (1997). "Language guiding therapy: the case of dehydration versus volume depletion". *Ann. Intern. Med.* 127 (9): 848–53. PMID 9382413. doi:10.7326/0003-4819-127-9-199711010-00020.

[112] Cancer. 1971 Jul;28(1):3-13., Epidemiology of cancer of the colon and rectum., Burkitt DP.

Several compounds of vegetable origin that our intestines are unable to absorb are classified as dietary fiber. They are therefore substances that never enter the bloodstream and cannot be used for energy production, cell growth or any chemical process. They never leave the intestines: the equivalent of landing in a city and never leaving the airport. Where does their importance come from, then?

Fibers help combat weight gain and obesity. Many studies[113] have analyzed and confirmed it, and the reasons are many: the fiber produces a feeling of satiety and leads to avoid eating compulsively; it limits the intake of fats and sugars by changing the composition of what passes through the intestine; it also seems to have an impact on weight gain.

A diet high in fiber lowers the glycemic index, as we have already seen, and therefore protects against type-two diabetes[114] and cardiovascular disease[115].

Fibers, as our friend Burkitt rightly noted, reduce the risk of colon cancer, probably due to the fact that their laxative effect decreases the average residence time of various waste in the intestine. In addition, the fibers induce some bacteria to produce a substance (butyric acid) that can protect against this disease[116].

More recent studies suggest a correlation between fiber intake and the decrease in other types of cancer: breast, prostate and digestive tract cancer. Many mechanisms still need to be clarified; for instance, the reduction in the risk of breast cancer seems to be linked to their ability to "cleanse" the body of some excess hormones (estrogens)[117].

---

[113] Nutrition. 2005 Mar;21(3):411-8., Dietary fiber and body weight., Slavin JL

[114] Diabetologia. 2015; 58(7): 1394–1408., Published online 2015 May 29. doi: 10.1007/s00125-015-3585-9, PMCID: PMC4472947, Dietary fibre and incidence of type 2 diabetes in eight European countries: the EPIC-InterAct Study and a meta-analysis of prospective studies, The InterAct Consortium

[115] Dietary fibre intake and risk of cardiovascular disease: systematic review and meta-analysis, *BMJ* 2013; 347 doi: https://doi.org/10.1136/bmj.f6879 (Published 19 December 2013)Cite this as: BMJ 2013;347:f6879, Diane E Threapleton, doctoral student, , Darren C Greenwood, senior lecturer in biostatistics, , Charlotte E L Evans, lecturer in nutritional epidemiology, , Christine L Cleghorn, research fellow, , Camilla Nykjaer, research assistant,, Charlotte Woodhead, research assistant, , Janet E Cade, professor of nutritional epidemiology group, , Christopher P Gale, associate professor of cardiovascular health sciences, Victoria J Burley, senior lecturer in nutritional epidemiology1

[116] Fuchs CS, Giovannucci EL, Colditz GA, et al. Dietary fiber and the risk of colorectal cancer and adenoma in women. *N Engl J Med*. 1999;340:169-176.

[117] Bagga D, Ashley JM, Geffrey SP, et al. Effects of a very low fat, high fiber diet on serum

The fibers, as the more constipated readers will know, have a laxative effect. This is due to their ability to absorb water: swelling in the intestine, they provide a volume of material that causes a mechanical stimulus whose effect is well known... This is provided (it is worth remembering) that you drink a lot.

Some types of fiber, as we will see better in the next paragraph, are the "food" of bacteria residing in the intestine that have extremely beneficial properties for us.

Fruits, vegetables and whole grains are rich in fiber. It is important that the daily diet ensures a sufficient amount of these elements. The diet we have described, which is rich in these foods, is perfect for this.

Before going any further: is anyone wondering what was Burkitt's second theory? Apparently, our fellow doctor had observed the natives really closely. According to Burkitt, the position with which many Africans at the time defecated (squatting, not sitting), had strong links with the reduced incidence of cancer. At the time the theory was buried because talking about that particular topic was strongly against common sensibility, but, out of curiosity, we can point out that some recent research seems to re-evaluate the relationship between the position in which one defecates and the health of the intestine. To do one's own physical needs in a crouching position, in particular, would apparently empty and cleanse the colon better... if you wish, you can then re-evaluate the pits in the garden that our great-grandfathers used...

The Incredible Experiment of Shy Mice

In 2011, the work team of Canadian researcher Stephen Collins conducted a rather strange experiment, one that might seem straight out of a science fiction tale. They took laboratory mice from two different strains with well-known behavioral characteristics: one shyer and more fearful; the other braver and more curious. They then gave them both a mix of antibiotics that erased their intestinal flora. Finally, they inoculated each strain with the bacteria that were in the intestines of the other.

hormones and menstrual function. Implications for breast cancer prevention. *Cancer*. 1999;76:2491-2496.

The two strains of mice reversed their behavioral characteristics: the brave ones became fearful, and vice versa. As if they were driven by the very bacteria that they housed inside[118]...

Each of us carries in our intestines a real world. Although it is difficult to imagine, there are more living beings within the belly of each of us than human beings on the entire planet.

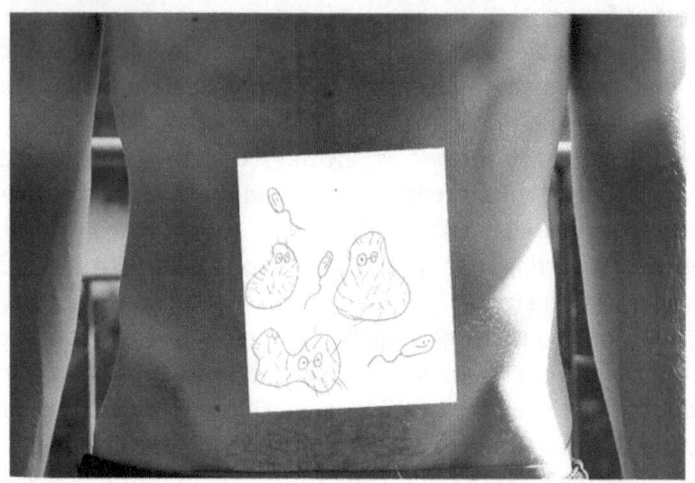

THE STRANGE GUESTS OF OUR INTESTINES ARE ESSENTIAL FOR OUR HEALTH. STRANGE BUT TRUE!

When we talk about intestinal flora, we refer in fact to the set of bacteria that populate our intestines. We are talking about millions of different species of microorganisms that have with us a symbiotic relationship. In symbiosis, different living beings live in close contact, and each of them is of benefit to the other.

What we give to the bacteria is clear: we allow them to feed themselves, in the warmth of our bowels, with the remains of our digestion. But what do they give us?

First, the bacteria present in the intestine carry out metabolic processes that our organism is not able to carry out autonomously. For instance, they can

[118] Gastroenterology. 2011 Aug;141(2):599-609, 609.e1-3. doi: 10.1053/j.gastro.2011.04.052. Epub 2011 Apr 30.

The intestinal microbiota affect central levels of brain-derived neurotropic factor and behavior in mice.

Bercik P1, Denou E, Collins J, Jackson W, Lu J, Jury J, Deng Y, Blennerhassett P, Macri J, McCoy KD, Verdu EF, Collins SM.

synthesize certain vitamins (folic acid, vitamin K, vitamins of the B group and others) and ferment the carbohydrates that remain from digestion to form a substance, butyric acid, which is the main source of energy for intestinal cells and, as we have seen, protects their mucous membranes.

In addition, intestinal bacteria living in symbiosis with us are in natural competition with harmful bacteria: in fact, they have every interest in ensuring that we, as host organisms, remain healthy. Colonies of "friendly" microorganisms therefore develop substances that are harmful to "enemy" microorganisms and, by multiplying, deprive them of the possibility of growing. Imagine being the mayor of a city besieged by youth gangs, and being allied with some of them, those that do not cause damage. "Friendly" gangs are the best way to counter vandalism in the area.

But the most recent research goes much further[119]: based on mechanisms still being investigated, the bacteria we host in our intestines may have a strong relationship with some chemical reactions that affect the well-being of our nervous system, and in particular the response to stress, anxiety and memory. These new frontiers of research may explain the strange experiment on rats mentioned at the beginning of this paragraph. And if we still don't know to what extent it can be comparable to what happens in humans, it is certain that the relationship between us and our bacteria is much more important than we thought in the past, and certainly vital.

What can we do to keep our guests healthy?

First, make sure that we often introduce new colonies of "good" bacteria with food, so that they can help existing ones and join them.

Most of the food we eat is low in bacteria; processed foods are, actually, sterile. Our ancestors, with their centuries-old culture, had learned the importance of periodically eating fermented foods that contain cultures of beneficial bacteria. In different parts of the world, there are recipes where different ingredients are brought to fermentation, for instance:

• Yoghurt (better if homemade, so the ferments remain fresh!) or its relative kefir: a drink from the Caucasus, rich in bacteria and healthy yeasts. Today, it can be found more and more in supermarkets

• The miso: a brown cream from the Far East, which is said to be one of the secrets of the strength of the Samurai. It comes from the fermentation of

[119] Ann Gastroenterol. 2015 Apr-Jun; 28(2): 203–209., PMCID: PMC4367209, The gut-brain axis: interactions between enteric microbiota, central and enteric nervous systems, Marilia Carabotti, Annunziata Scirocco, Maria Antonietta Maselli and Carola Severi

cereals such as soya and rice, and gives great benefits to the intestinal flora in a short time

•   From northern Europe sauerkraut: fermented cabbages that develop cultures of beneficial bacteria within them. In addition to cabbage, many other vegetables can be fermented, such as onions, olives, cucumbers, carrots, peppers, apples, turnips....

Adding these foods, from time to time, to our diet, is certainly very beneficial to the health of the intestine and the entire body. A pioneering study shows the benefits of fermented foods on the physical and mental health of the body, as our ancestors have known for thousands of years[120].

In addition, we can undoubtedly do good to our intestinal flora by regularly taking substances on which it feeds. Once again, we are talking about indigestible fibers, referred to as prebiotics, which form the basis of the sustenance of intestinal bacteria. The foods richest in prebiotics are nuts, roots, fruit peel and whole grains. Once again, a varied diet based on food as found in nature is the key to well-being from every point of view.

---

[120] J Physiol Anthropol. 2014; 33(1): 2.Published online 2014 Jan 15. doi: 10.1186/1880-6805-33-2, PMCID: PMC3904694, Fermented foods, microbiota, and mental health: ancient practice meets nutritional psychiatry, Eva M Selhub, Alan C Logan, and Alison C Bested

Conclusions

The book *Babette's Feast* by Karen Blixen tells of a couple of old puritan sisters living in a Norwegian fjord, who have dedicated their lives to their neighbor, giving up one to love and the other to the career as an opera singer.

One day, Babette, a French fugitive in search of asylum sent by an acquaintance, shows up at their house. Babette becomes the housekeeper of the sisters, and earns the respect and admiration of the whole village.

Several years later, Babette inherits a large sum of money, which everyone believes she will use to return to France to spend a comfortable life. To celebrate, the housekeeper organizes a lunch for the whole village, having fine and exclusive food arrive from France on purpose and cooking a luxury restaurant menu (Babette was in fact a chef before fleeing): turtle broth, Dermidoff blinis (crepes of Russian origin), quails in puff pastry, savarin with fresh fruit, along with vintage wines.

Puritan Norwegians, accustomed to a life of deprivation and renunciation, are literally inebriated by Babette's lunch, so much so as to live almost a mystical experience, outside the limits imposed by their vision of life.

To buy the ingredients and get them into that remote fjord, however, Babette spends all the money of the inheritance. Only the old general, the old love of one of the two sisters, can understand, incredulously, the real value of that lunch. Babette renounces to rebuild her life to thank the community who welcomed her, and in doing so gives birth, from her sacrifice, to a new sense of existence for all.

We are literally made by what we swallow, and the choice of food is an act of respect towards our body, a gift that we give to ourselves as important and magical as the one Babette gives to her community.

We have reached the end of this journey. We hope to have been able to illustrate interesting concepts without having bored you to death. Most of all, we hope to have conveyed a very clear message: human nutrition is a science, and as such should be treated. As you have seen, everything we ingest triggers very specific chemical reactions on which the functioning of our bodies and our well-being depend.

Following a diet read in a weekly magazine or recommended by a friend is therefore not a decision to be taken lightly; we believe that we have given you the tools to create autonomously a varied, balanced and healthy diet, not dependent on the food fashions of the moment or on what the industry wants you to believe. A diet that (provided you have a medical consent for it), can simply make you feel good, maximizing your energy and health levels or, if you need it, help you achieve your goals in terms of weight loss (or gain).

Furthermore, we hope that we have conveyed curiosity about the world of food and its effects, and that the rich bibliography of this book can be a starting point for discovering and learning.

Finally, we hope that we have properly emphasized that real, genuine, unprocessed food is the only one that must be taken into consideration. Always remember: Mother Nature is not stupid, and a rich, healthy and balanced diet always starts from what it provides us with, as it is. Stay away from fashions and excesses, rediscover the taste of the foods that your great-grandmother would have cooked ... in a few months, you will have the pleasure of being renewed and fitter, more beautiful and happier.

Good luck, and that you too may receive Babette's gift!

Appendix A - Vitamins: Effects, Symptoms of Deficiency, Foods That Are Rich in Them

Vitamin A (retinol): It is essential for the growth and health of many organs of our body: the mucous membranes, lungs, digestive system, skin, bones, teeth and blood circulation. It also has regulatory effects on sleep and blood pressure. Its deficiency causes eye problems (up to a reduction in visual intensity), reduced resistance to infections, nervousness, anxiety and migraine. Vitamin A deficiency is the leading cause of childhood blindness in poorer countries.

Foods rich in this vitamin are: cod liver oil, liver, egg yolk, butter, raw carrots, garlic, spinach, cabbage, parsley, wheat germ oil, dandelion, watercress, tomato, broccoli, potatoes, mango, chicory, lettuce, pumpkin, apricots, melon, peach, orange, watermelon, generally all yellow or orange fruits. Attention: coffee, alcohol, tobacco, cortisone and antibiotics decrease or neutralize the absorption of vitamin A.

Vitamin D (in its two forms, cholecalciferol and ergocalciferol): It is the exception to the general rule by which we cannot produce the vitamins we need ourselves. This vitamin, in fact, is produced by our skin when it is hit by the sun's rays. Especially in the Nordic countries or in the winter months; in fact, it is a substance of which it is extremely easy to be deficient. In the past, rachitic children were exposed to ultraviolet light to allow them to supplement this vitamin, which is essential for bone growth and development, but also for nerve and heart health. Its deficiency is linked to bone disorders such as rickets and osteoporosis; it is also associated with anemia and rheumatism.

It is more difficult to take with food; it is present in some fish (such as salmon and herring), cod liver oil, eggs, liver and green vegetables.

Vitamin E (tocopherol): It is associated with the health of the red blood cells and the fluidization of the blood; it also plays an important role in slowing down the aging process. Its deficiency, which is quite rare, causes anemia and problems with the reproductive system (sterility in men and ease of abortion in women).

It is found mainly in vegetable oils (olive, seeds, corn...) of sunflowers, dried fruit, milk and its derivatives, basil, spinach, turnip greens, potatoes, mango and avocado.

Vitamin K: It is essential for the coagulation of blood, that is, the reaction that allows the blood to "patch" the wounds. Its deficiency therefore causes hemorrhages. It is also synthesized by the bacteria inhabiting our intestines, so its deficiency is quite rare.

Food sources: green leafy vegetables, chickpeas, peas, soya, green tea, eggs, liver, dairy products and meat.

Vitamin B1 (thiamine): In addition to regulating the metabolism of carbohydrates, it facilitates digestion, helps heart health and is essential for growth. It is also extremely beneficial for the nervous system and its efficiency. Deficiency causes tiredness, headaches, memory problems, irritability, dizziness and lack of appetite. In extreme conditions of deficiency, a disease known as beriberi develops, which can result in paralysis.

The following foods are rich in it: whole grains, pork, innards, brewer's yeast, legumes, oranges, pineapple and melon.

Vitamin B2 (riboflavin): It regulates the intestinal balance and, at the cellular level, the metabolism of sugars, fats and proteins. Deficiency causes gastrointestinal disorders, skin, eye and mucous membrane damage, cramps and tiredness.

Foods rich in it are yeast, milk, innards, egg white, all cereals, especially wholemeal cereals, algae, spinach, potatoes, mushrooms, almonds and bananas.

Vitamin B3 (or PP, or niacin): It is an important factor in metabolism, rebalances the nervous system by acting as an antidepressant and is also important for the circulation. Its deficiency causes pellagra, a terrible disease that causes dermatitis, dementia, diarrhea and skin flaking, and that was widespread among farmers in past centuries, when food was almost exclusively enough on corn, poor in this substance.

We can find it in all cereals, especially wholemeal ones, mushrooms, potatoes, avocado, peanuts, brewer's yeast and in most meats.

Vitamin B5 (pantothenic acid): it is important for the prevention of infections, the reduction of tiredness and stress and the health of skin and hair. Its lack can lead to forms, even very severe, of loss of sensitivity of the limbs (paresthesia).

Very common in food, and in particular in most vegetables and also in liver, brewer's yeast, wheat bran, sesame seeds, royal jelly, sunflower seeds, soya, eggs, dried peas, buckwheat wholemeal flour and legumes.

Vitamin B6 (pyridoxine): It allows the assimilation of proteins by the body and is indispensable for the production of antibodies and red blood cells. Its deficiency causes anemia and disorders of the nervous system.

We find it in all whole grains, potatoes, tomatoes, spinach, avocado, bananas, melons and oranges. Also present in dairy products, fish and meat.

Biotin: This is the vitamin with the most names; depending on countries and times it has been called vitamin B7, B8, I or H. Regardless of its name, it remains essential for the proper functioning of the liver and immune system; it is also important for the nervous system and fat metabolism. Its deficiency causes dermatitis and intestinal disorders.

Present mainly in milk and dairy products, eggs, seafood, legumes, cereals, almonds, spinach and mushrooms.

Vitamin B9 (folic acid): It is involved in the formation of red blood cells and in the synthesis of amino acids. Its deficiency causes depression, apathy, insomnia, anxiety. It is essential during pregnancy, because in its absence the unborn child may have malformations of the nervous system.

Offal, green leafy vegetables, eggs, legumes, oranges, asparagus and broccoli are some of the foods richer in it.

Vitamin B12 (cobalamin): Essential for the formation of red and white blood cells; it also promotes growth and protects the nervous system by improving concentration and memory. Its deficiency causes anemia.

It is mainly present in products of animal origin (meat, fish, dairy products, eggs), and in some algae.

Vitamin C (ascorbic acid): It is essential for the formation of collagen and strengthens the immune system. It also has other functions: for instance, it helps to fix calcium on the bones, improves the absorption of minerals and other vitamins. Its deficiency causes scurvy.

All citrus fruits, peppers and chilies, rocket, broccoli, kiwi, lettuce, Brussels sprouts, strawberries, broad beans, peas, tomatoes and papayas are rich in it.

Appendix B - Mineral Salts: Effects, Symptoms of Deficiency, Foods That Are Rich in Them

Calcium: Essential for the growth and maintenance of bones and teeth; also necessary for muscle contraction, blood clotting and the transmission of nerve impulses. Milk and dairy products, eggs, legumes and fish are rich in it. Its deficiency causes bone diseases such as rickets and osteoporosis as well as tetanus crises.

Phosphorus: It is widespread in bone tissue and teeth and is also present in muscle tissue and blood. In addition to playing a key role in energy production, it is essential to bones, teeth and muscles. Milk, cheese, meat, fish and legumes are all rich in it. Deficiency causes weakness and demineralization of bones.

Magnesium: Used by bone, nerve and muscle tissue. It is found in nuts, hazelnuts, cocoa, tea leaves, almonds, and some spices. Its deficiency is associated with anorexia, vomiting and increased muscle excitability.

Sodium: Fundamental for the life of cells, in that it regulates the exchanges between them and the outside together with potassium. Contained in cooking salt, cheese and sausages. The deficiency is responsible for anorexia, nausea and vomiting, but a quantity of more than 4 grams/0.1 ounce may lead to hypertension.

Potassium: Together with sodium, as seen above, it is fundamental for cellular exchanges. Beans, peas, spinach, asparagus, potatoes and bananas are all rich in it. Deficiency causes muscle cramps and abnormal heart rhythms.

Chlorine: It is involved in the digestion process at the gastric level. It is bound to sodium in cooking salt. Its deficiency causes muscle cramps.

Sulfur: It is essential for the growth of hair, nails and cartilage. Sulfur is present in animal proteins.

Iron: Essential for the functioning of red blood cells, which allow to bring oxygen to the cells of our body and to clean them of carbon dioxide. Present in fish, eggs, spinach and meat. Iron deficiency causes asthenia and anemia.

Copper: Associated with the proper functioning of the heart, kidneys and brain. Contained in liver, legumes, crustaceans and wheat germ. Its deficiency causes bone fragility and anemia.

Zinc: It contributes to the initiation of many chemical reactions in our organism. Meat, cocoa, egg yolk and nuts are all rich in it. Deficiency can cause a variety of symptoms, such as delays in wound healing and immune response, skin changes, hypogonadism and dwarfism.

Fluorine: Important for the growth and maintenance of bones and teeth, it is mainly assumed through drinking water. Deficiency is a major factor in facilitating dental caries.

Iodine: Indispensable for the formation of hormones produced by the thyroid. Algae, iodized salt and mollusks are rich in iodine. The deficiency causes the typical "goiter", with tiredness, depression, cysts and weight gain.

Selenium: It protects cell membranes from free radicals and is thought to have an anti-aging function. The main sources are cereals and meat. Deficiency causes heart and liver disorders.

Chromium: It contributes to the physiological metabolism of fats and sugars. It abounds in brewer's yeast, wheat, carrots, black pepper and peas. The deficiency causes an increase in glycemia, triglycerides and cholesterol.

Cobalt: It is associated with the formation of vitamin B12. Contained mainly in meat, dairy products and seafood, its deficiency causes anemia.

Manganese: Important for growth, it is involved in numerous chemical reactions and has an antioxidant function. Cereals and nuts are rich in it. Its deficiency causes a slowdown in growth and can facilitate diabetes.

Molybdenum: It is present in the liver and kidneys, and is important for many metabolic reactions. It abounds in offal, legumes and cereals. The deficiency is linked to irritability and tachycardia.

Appendix C - The Different Types of Fats in Some Foods (Indicative Average Compositions)

Goose and duck fat: 35% saturated fat, 52% monounsaturated fat, 13% polyunsaturated fat. Proportion of omega-6 and omega-3 fatty acids: depends on animal feed.

Chicken fat: 31% saturated fat, 49% monounsaturated fat, 20% polyunsaturated fat. Proportion of omega-6 and omega-3 fatty acids: mostly omega6; omega3s are higher in organic chickens.

Lard or pig fat: 40% saturated fat, 48% monounsaturated, 12% polyunsaturated. Proportion of omega-6 and omega-3 fatty acids: depends on animal feed.

Beef fat: 50-55% saturated fat, 40% monounsaturated, small amounts of polyunsaturated.

Olive oil: 75%, monounsaturated, 13% saturated, 10% omega-6 polyunsaturated, 2% omega-3 polyunsaturated.

Peanut oil: 48% monounsaturated; 18% saturated; 34% omega-6 polyunsaturated.

Sesame oil: 42% unsaturated, 15% saturated; 43% omega-6 polyunsaturated.

Corn, soya, sunflower, cotton seed oil: More than 50% omega-6 polyunsaturated.

Rapeseed oil: 5% saturated fat, 57% monounsaturated, 23% omega-6 polyunsaturated; 10% -15% omega-3 polyunsaturated.

Linseed oil: 9% saturated, 18% unsaturated, 16% omega-6 polyunsaturated; 57% omega-3 polyunsaturated.

Palm oil: 50% saturated fat, 41% monounsaturated, 9% omega-6 polyunsaturated.

Coconut oil: 92% saturated.

Appendix D - Index and Glycemic Load (per 100 grams/3.5 ounces of Each Food) of the Main Foods

The first number is the glycemic index; the second number is the glycemic load per 100 grams/3.5 ounces.

Fruit

avocado 10-0

black cherry 22-2

cherry 25-4

strawberry 25-1

raspberry 25-2

blueberries 25-1

blackberry 25-2

blackcurrant 25-2

apricot 30-2

clementine 30-3

mandarin 30-5

pear 30-3

grapefruit 30-2

orange 35-3

coconut 35-3

fig 35-4

apple 35-4

Pomegranate 35-6

Fishing 35-2

Plum 35-4

Pineapple 45-5

Grapes 45-8

Kiwi 50-5

Litchi 50-9

Mango 50-6

Papaya 55-4

Banana 60-9

Watermelon 75-6

Melon 75-6

legumes

Peanuts 14-1

lentils cooked 25-4

cooked peas 25-5

soy milk 30-0

boiled chickpeas 30-8

cooked beans 35-4

raw beans 40-2

Cereals

Muesli 65-57

corn flakes 81-104

bran cereals 38-37

raw oat bran 15-10

wheat bran 15-4

barley beans 25-16

oatmeal 30-3

whole wheat barley flour 30-24

cooked amaranth 35-7

Quinoa cooked 35-9

raw oat flakes 40-27

buckwheat in grains 40-25

couscous 50-72

oatmeal 45-33

buckwheat flour 45-28

integral basmati rice 45-23

rye in grains 45-29

wholemeal rye flour 45-29

cooked brown rice 50-13

whole wheat flour 60-38

whole wheat flour 60-41

barley beans 60-42

cooked pearl barley 60-17

whole wheat flour 65-44

Corn 65 -49

Amaranth 70-46

cornmeal 70-57

Millet 70-51

wheat flour 0 85-65

wheat flour 00 85-66

corn starch 85-74

boiled parboiled rice 85-20

puffed rice 85-72

rice milk 85-8

tapioca 85-81

rice flour 95-83

Sweeteners:

stevia 0 -0

saccharin 0-0

sucralose 0-0

cyclamate o 0-0

Aspartame 0-0

Acesulfame 0-0

agave syrup 15-11

fructose 20-20

galactose 25-25

maltitol 35-0

apple juice 50-6

maple syrup 65-44

white sugar 70-73

raw cane sugar 70-73

Molasses 70-52

Honey 85-68

Maltodextrin 85-80

wheat malt 100-71

glucose syrup 100-100

Maltose 105-105

Protein foods

Eggs 0-0

Meat 0-0

Fish 0-0

Cheese 0-0

unsweetened low-fat yogurt 20-1

whole yogurt 53-2

skim milk 47-2

Pasta, Bread and Pizza

whole wheat flour bread with sourdough 40-19

unleavened bread with whole wheat flour 40-35

whole grain buckwheat bread 40-34

wholemeal pasta 40-12

pasta 40-12

whole wheat rye bread 45-20

kamut bread 45-27

Pizza (dough) 60-44

pizza margherita (all) 80-22

white bread 70-56

loaf of bread 85-57

hamburger bread 85--76

crackers 70-76

Snack

ice cream 60-18

orange juice 52-33

chocolate bar 65-34

milk chocolate 44-35

French fries 70-36

croissant 67-43

jam 40-44

pastries 53-54

biscuits 61-63

wafers 77-85

vegetables

Beetroot 65-4

Pumpkin 75-4

raw carrots 30-5

cooked carrots 85-5

boiled white potato 70 -14

The values refer to the portion indicated and shall be considered as indicative, as they may vary depending on factors such as, for instance, the degree of ripeness of the fruit, the methods of preparation/baking, ingredients, brands for industrial products, etc.

How to calculate the amount of food to be taken so that the glycemic load is equal to ten:

Let C be the glycemic load, I be the glycemic index, Q1 be the amount of carbohydrates in 100 grams/3.5 ounces of food and Q2 be the amount of food we need to derive.

From the definition of glycemic load, we have C= (I x Q1) /100, hence Q1= (100 x C) /I.

Replacing in the definition 10 to C, we obtain 10= (I x Q1) /100, from which Q1=1000/I, that is to say to have the load equal to ten, it is necessary that the quantity of carbohydrates taken is equal to one thousand divided by the glycemic index.

To find out how much total food corresponds to this condition, let's structure this proportion between the carbohydrates in 100 grams/3.5 ounces of food (Q1 by definition) and those (equal to 1000/I) in the final amount of food Q2:

(1000/I): Q2 = Q1: 100

Replacing in this proportion to Q1 the expression (100 x C) /I obtained at the beginning, and then obtaining Q2, we have Q2=1000/C

Appendix E - Calories (Kcal) per 100 grams/3.5 ounces of Food

Foods are in alphabetical order for easy reference.
The value indicated refers to Kcal per 100 grams/3.5 ounces of food.

Almonds 576
Anchovy 101
Apple 54
Apricot 47
Artichoke 22
Asparagus 18
Avocado 223
Bacon 854
Baguette 270
Banana 94
Beer 47
Beetroot 41
Blackcurrant 33
Blueberries 38
Bresaola 128
Brie 315
Broccoli 27
Butter 754
Camembert 281
Carp 115
Carpaccio 121
Carrot 27
Cauliflower 23
Celery 15
Champagne 83
Cherry 59
Chestnuts 196
Chicken breast 114
chicken broth 257
Chicken sausage 173

Chickpeas 275
Chop (mutton) 348
Chop (pork) 150
Chop (veal) 112
Coconut oil 895
Coconut pulp 369
Cod 73
Cooked ham 193
Corn 333
Corn starch 346
Cucumber 13
Custard 122
Dates 273
Duck 227
Egg (whole) 159
Eggplant 17
Emmental 387
Escalope (pork) 106
Escalope (veal) 100
Fennel 24
Fig 60
Fillet (beef) 121
Fillet (pork) 106
Fillet (veal) 95
Fish 47
Fresh cheese 253
Fructose 290
Full fat milk 47
Garlic 135
Goat cheese 355
Goat cheese 219
Goose 342
Gorgonzola cheese 358
Grapefruit 43
Grapefruit juice 36
Grapes (dried) 276
Grapes (fresh) 73

Green beans 35
Ground beef 216
Ground pork 271
Hake 91
Hazelnuts 643
Herring 193
Honey 325
Kiwi 50
Lard 900
Leek 26
Lemon 36
Lentils 310
Liver 121
Lobster 84
Mackerel 180
Mango 56
Maple syrup 270
Margarine 722
Mayonnaise 752
Melon 54
Melted butter 900
Mortadella 345
Mozzarella 255
Muesli 394
Mushrooms (dried) 124
Mushrooms (fresh) 17
Mussels 51
Nuts 667
Oat flakes 354
Olive oil 900
Olives 351
Onion 28
Orange 44
Orange juice 47
Oysters 66
Palm oil 894
Parmesan cheese 386

Pasta 137
Peanuts 571
Pear 55
Peas 272
Pepper 20
Pike 82
Pineapple 57
Pistachios 598
Plum (dried) 236
Plum (fresh) 51
Pork sausage 298
Pork shank 100
Potato 71
Potato starch 336
Pumpkin 25
Pumpkin seeds 570
Radishes 13
Raspberries 32
Raspberry 44
Raw ham 383
Rice 116
Roast 161
Roast chicken 166
Salami 232
Salmon (fresh) 202
Salmon (smoked) 289
Sardines 124
Savoy 25
Shrimp 87
Skimmed milk 35
Soft cheese 374
Sole 83
Soybean 323
Spaghetti 145
Spinach (fresh) 15
Sprouts 38
Strawberry 33

Striploin   130
Sugar   410
Swordfish   117
Thigh (beef)   148
Thigh (chicken)   174
Thigh (pork)   274
Thigh (veal)   97
Tomato   17
Trout   102
Truffle   56
Tuna   226
Turkey breast   212
Veal sausage   266
Vodka   222
Watermelon   38
Wheat bran   176
Wheat semolina   324
Whiskey   438
White beans   262
White bread   238
Whole corn flour   333
Wholemeal wheat bread   200
Wine (red)   69
Wine (white)   69
Yoghurt (low fat)   34
Yoghurt (natural)   46
Yolk   68

Disclaimer

This book is intended as a mere integration to the advice of qualified health professionals, not as a replacement. Always consult a doctor before starting any diet. Author and publisher disclaim any responsibility for consequences arising from the application of any content of this work.

Credit information for the images

Proteins and Amino Acids:
- bowels: from the book "The Human Body and Health Revised", Alvin Davison, public domain image

Vitamins and Mineral Salts:
- collagen fibres: Scanning electron microscopy of collagen fibres. Credit: Tom Deerinck and Mark Ellisman, NCMIR: license: https://creativecommons.org/licenses/by/2.0/legalcode
- Soil: Terreno arado para plantação REFON 1.JPG, author: Jose Reynaldo da Fonseca
- Vegetables: credit: Rick Ligthelm. License: https://creativecommons.org/licenses/by/2.0/legalcode

Carbohydrates:
- Bread: picture by Sandstein, released under Creative Commons Attribution 3.0 Unported

Let's take a First Stock of the Situation
- Fast food meal: picture by LukeB20161933
- Convenience store: picture by AlejandroLinaresGarcia

Enzymes and Hormones:
- Little baby with saliva on his lips: image by Pereru, Creative Commons Attribution-Share Alike 4.0 International license, https://upload.wikimedia.org/wikipedia/commons/5/5d/Saliva_Baby.jpg
- Red geranium petal cells: image by Umberto Salvagnin, https://www.flickr.com/photos/kaibara/4966621857, Creative Common License CC BY 2.0

The Metabolism of Carbohydrates:
- SPA signboard: "Relaxing Massage Unisex Salon By Monic" by Monic Massage, modified. Creative Common Attribution 2.0 Generic: https://creativecommons.org/licenses/by/2.0/legalcode. Original image: https://www.flickr.com/photos/monic_massage/14669384445

The Metabolism of Fats:
- Cake: by Toby Oxborrow from Kowloon, Hong Kong, released under the Creative Commons Attribution-Share Alike 2.0 Generic license.
- Muscle tissue: photo by Department of Histology, Jagiellonian University Medical College, released under Creative Commons Attribution-Share Alike 3.0 Unported
- "wanted" signs: by radtasticbxtch, "wanted poster" released under Creative Commons License, attribution 2.0 generic (CC BY2.0). Changes have been made, substituting the face inside the posters with other images.
- Cigarette: "a lit cigarette in an ashtray" by Tomasz Sienicki, released under Creative Commons Attribution-Share Alike 3.0 Unported license

The metabolism of proteins:
- Manneken Pis: by PMRMaeyaert, released under the under the Creative Commons Attribution-Share Alike 3.0 Unported license.

Insulin and glucagon:

- Girl eating: photo by Alpha, "Julia eating giant Roast Beef Baguette - Pub Bistro, Thredbo", released under the Creative Commons Attribution-ShareAlike 2.0 Generic (CC BY-SA 2.0)
- Muscle tissue: "diagram of muscle cells" by Cancer Research UK, licensed under the Creative Commons Attribution-Share Alike 4.0 International license.
- Man and woman running: Chris Hunkeler, "Running Styles", released under the Attribution-ShareAlike 2.0 Generic (CC BY-SA 2.0)
- Pasta: "Pasta with pesto" by Paul Goyette, released under the Creative Commons Attribution-Share Alike 2.0 Generic license.

The right composition of the diet:

- Vegetables inside Harvard's plate: "Fresh herbs, fresh spices and vegetables sold at a stall in Thanin Market, Chiang Mai, Thailand" by Takeaway, released under the Creative Commons Attribution-Share Alike 3.0 Unported license.
- Fruits inside Harvard's plate: "Common culinary fruits. Bananas, apples, pears, strawberries, oranges, grapes, canary melons, water melon, cantaloupe, pineapple and mango. Picture by Bill Ebbesen" by Ionutzmovie, licensed under the Creative Commons Attribution 3.0 Unported license.
- Grains inside Harvard's plate: "Wheat grains kept for drying at Madhurawada, Visakhapatnam, India" by Adityamadhav83, released under Creative Commons Attribution-Share Alike 3.0 Unported license
- Protein foods inside Harvard's plate: "A range of protein-rich foods" by Smastronardo, licensed under the Creative Commons Attribution-Share Alike 4.0 International license

Calories and body weight:

- lightning: "An image of pink lightning taken during a storm" by oompa123; source: http://oompa123.deviantart.com/art/lightning-last-year-168039966, released under the Creative Commons Attribution 3.0 Unported license.
- weight scale : "Simple laboratory scales for balancing tubes" by Lilly_M, licensed under the Creative Commons Attribution-Share Alike 3.0 Unported, 2.5 Generic, 2.0 Generic and 1.0 Generic license.

Summary